Functional Neurosurgery

NEUROSURGERY BY EXAMPLE

Key Cases and Fundamental Principles
Series edited by: Nathan R. Selden, MD, PhD, FACS, FAAP

Functional Neurosurgery

Edited by

Ahmed M. Raslan
Ashwin Viswanathan

OXFORD
UNIVERSITY PRESS

Oxford University Press is a department of the University of Oxford. It furthers
the University's objective of excellence in research, scholarship, and education
by publishing worldwide. Oxford is a registered trade mark of Oxford University
Press in the UK and certain other countries.

Published in the United States of America by Oxford University Press
198 Madison Avenue, New York, NY 10016, United States of America.

Library of Congress Control Number: 2019031807
ISBN 978–0–19–088762–9

This material is not intended to be, and should not be considered, a substitute for medical or other professional advice. Treatment for the conditions described in this material is highly dependent on the individual
circumstances. And, while this material is designed to offer accurate information with respect to the subject
matter covered and to be current as of the time it was written, research and knowledge about medical and
health issues is constantly evolving and dose schedules for medications are being revised continually, with new
side effects recognized and accounted for regularly. Readers must therefore always check the product information
and clinical procedures with the most up-to-date published product information and data sheets provided by the
manufacturers and the most recent codes of conduct and safety regulation. The publisher and the authors make
no representations or warranties to readers, express or implied, as to the accuracy or completeness of this material.
Without limiting the foregoing, the publisher and the authors make no representations or warranties as to the
accuracy or efficacy of the drug dosages mentioned in the material. The authors and the publisher do not accept,
and expressly disclaim, any responsibility for any liability, loss or risk that may be claimed or incurred as a conse-
quence of the use and/or application of any of the contents of this material.

9 8 7 6 5 4 3 2 1

Printed by Integrated Books International, United States of America

Contents

Series Editor's Preface

Dear Reader,

I am delighted to introduce this volume in the series *Neurosurgery by Example: Key Cases and Fundamental Principles*. Neurosurgical training and practice are based on managing a wide range of complex clinical cases with expert knowledge, sound judgment, and skilled technical execution. Our goal in this series is to present exemplary cases in the manner they are actually encountered in the neurosurgical clinic, hospital emergency department, and operating room.

For this volume, Drs. Ahmed Raslan and Ashwin Viswanathan invited a broad range of expert contributors to share their extensive wisdom and experience in all major areas of functional neurosurgery. Each chapter contains a classic presentation of an important clinical entity, guiding readers through the assessment and planning, decision-making, surgical procedure, aftercare, and complication management. "Pivot points" illuminate the changes required to manage patients in alternate or atypical situations.

Each chapter also presents lists of pearls for the accurate diagnosis, successful treatment, and effective complication management of each clinical problem. These three focus areas will be especially helpful to neurosurgeons preparing to sit for the American Board of Neurological Surgery oral examination, which bases scoring on these three topics.

Finally, each chapter contains focused reviews of medical evidence and expected outcomes, helpful for counseling patients and setting accurate expectations. Rather than exhaustive reference lists, chapter authors provide focused lists of high-priority additional reading recommended to deepen understanding.

The resulting volume should provide you with a dynamic tour through the practice of functional neurosurgery guided by some of the leading experts in North America. Additional volumes cover each subspecialty area of neurosurgery, using the same case-based approach and board review features.

Nathan R. Selden, MD, PhD
Campagna Professor and Chair
Department of Neurological Surgery
Oregon Health & Science University

Contributors

Walid A. Abdel Ghany, MD, PhD
Professor of Neurological Surgery
Ain Shams University
Cairo, Egypt

Daniel J. Curry, MD
The John S. Dunn Foundation Endowed
    Chair for Minimally Invasive Epilepsy
    Surgery, Texas Children's Hospital
Director, Functional Neurosurgery &
    Epilepsy Surgery, Texas Children's
    Hospital
Associate Professor, Department of
    Neurosurgery
Baylor College of Medicine
Houston, TX, USA

Nisha Giridharan, MD
Neurosurgery Resident
Department of Neurosurgery
Baylor College of Medicine
Houston, TX, USA

Casey H. Halpern, MD
Assistant Professor in Neurological
    Surgery
Stanford University
Palo Alto, CA, USA

Allen L. Ho, MD
Department of Neurological Surgery
Stanford University
Palo Alto, CA, USA

Christian Hoelscher, MD
Department of Neurological Surgery
Thomas Jefferson University
Philadelphia, PA, USA

Patrick J. Karas, MD
Neurosurgery Resident
Department of Neurosurgery
Baylor College of Medicine
Houston, TX, USA

Michael Kinsman, MD
Assistant Professor in Neurological
    Surgery
University of Kansas Medical Center
Lawrence, KS, USA

Kelly Layton, PA-C
Department of Neurological Surgery
Thomas Jefferson University
Philadelphia, PA, USA

Jonathan P. Miller, MD, FAANS, FACS
Professor of Neurological Surgery
University Hospitals Case
    Medical Center
Cleveland, OH, USA

Mohamed A. Nada, MD
Consultant of Neurosurgery
Department of Neurosurgery
Ministry of Health
Dar Elshefaa Hospital
Cairo, Egypt

Thomas Ostergard, MD, MS
Department of Neurological Surgery
University Hospitals Case
    Medical Center
Cleveland, OH, USA

Ahmed M. Raslan, MBBCh, MSc, MD
Associate Professor of Neurological
 Surgery
Oregon Health & Science University
Portland, OR, USA

Gaddum Duemani Reddy, MD, PhD
Department of Neurological Surgery
Upstate Medical University
Syracuse, NY, USA

Jonathan Riley, MD
Assistant Professor in Neurological
 Surgery
State University of New York at Buffalo
Buffalo, NY, USA

Mariah Sami, MD
Department of Neurological Surgery
University of Kansas
Lawrence, KS, USA

Richard Schmidt, MD, PhD
Department of Neurological Surgery
Thomas Jefferson University
Philadelphia, PA, USA

**Nathan R. Selden, MD, PhD, FACS,
 FAAP**
Campagna Professor and Chair
Department of Neurological Surgery
Oregon Health & Science University
Portland, OR, USA

Kyle Smith, MD
Department of Neurological Surgery
University of Kansas
Lawrence, KS, USA

Zoe E. Teton
Department of Neurological
 Surgery
Oregon Health & Science
 University
Portland, OR, USA

Ashwin Viswanathan, MD
Associate Professor in Neurological
 Surgery
Baylor College of Medicine
Houston, TX, USA

Chengyuan Wu, MD, MSBME
Assistant Professor in Neurological
 Surgery
Thomas Jefferson University
Philadelphia, PA, USA

Stephanie Zyck, MD
Department of Neurological
 Surgery
Upstate Medical University
Syracuse, NY, USA

Functional Neurosurgery

Bilateral Essential Tremor

Kelly Layton, Jonathan Riley, Richard Schmidt,
Christian Hoelscher, and Chengyuan Wu

Case Presentation

The patient is a 60-year-old gentleman with an 8-year history of worsening tremor in both hands, with resultant difficulty completing manual tasks, particularly those that involve fine motor function. He also notes progressive difficulty with activities of daily living (ADL), including eating, drinking, writing, and typing. The patient is a professional golfer and states that the tremor has now progressed to the point that he is unable to play. He has no symptoms at rest, states that his tremor begins at movement onset, and worsens when his arms are outstretched. The tremor affects his left hand to a greater degree than his right hand. He does report some mild tremor with his head, although this symptom started relatively recently. He reports that both his mother and his brother were previously diagnosed with essential tremor. He denies any other neurological complaints and any history of psychiatric or behavioral comorbidities. The patient does occasionally drink alcohol and states that doing so sometimes helps his tremor.

The patient is a well-appearing man for his stated age. He exhibits a normal affect, is able to converse normally, and does not have any speech, cognitive, or memory deficits. Cranial nerves are grossly intact. Motor strength is 5/5 throughout all muscle groups, and sensation and deep tendon reflexes are normal. The patient exhibits normal gait with no ataxia and has normal rapid alternating movements with no dysmetria. The patient has a significant intention tremor with purposeful movement in both of his hands, left greater than right. The tremor was low amplitude with a frequency about 6 Hz; however, the tremor increased in amplitude when his arms were outstretched.

Questions

1. What is the differential diagnosis of a patient with this presentation?
2. What components of the patient's history or physical examination suggest the suspected diagnosis? What key parts of the history or physical examination separate it from other diseases on the differential diagnosis?
3. Is there a familial inheritance of this disorder? What about a specific gene?
4. What is the initial management in this condition? What would suggest surgical intervention as a possible option in this patient?
5. What imaging is needed prior to intervention?

Assessment and Planning

The patient has been under the care of a neurologist, who initially prescribed propranolol for the patient's essential tremor. Although the patient initially demonstrated some response, his symptoms returned, and he was subsequently treated with primidone and lorazepam on an as needed basis. Despite medication, the patient's symptoms progressively worsened. As such, he was referred for evaluation for possible deep brain stimulation (DBS). After thorough medical evaluation, the patient was determined to be a safe surgical candidate. Risks and benefits of surgical intervention were discussed at length with the patient and his family, and he is scheduled for DBS.

Questions

1. What is the primary surgical target for the treatment of essential tremor?
2. What are the different surgical options for the treatment of essential tremor? What intraoperative adjuncts exist to help with surgical planning and electrode placement?

Oral Boards Review—Diagnostic Pearls

1. Essential tremor is associated with movement, and the worst tremor occurs with arms outstretched. There is typically no resting tremor, although a slight subtle tremor may be seen with progressive disease.
2. The tremor is typically bilateral and located in the upper extremities; however, symptoms may be slightly lateralized to the dominant side. Tremor may occasionally be seen in the head or neck, especially in progressive disease. Unilateral symptoms and isolated head or leg tremors raise concern for an alternate diagnosis.
3. The tremor is typically the only presenting neurological symptom, although some mild rigidity may be observed. Any other neurological finding, especially dysmetria, cogwheel rigidity, cognitive or behavioral abnormalities, or focal weakness, should raise consideration of an alternative diagnosis.

Decision-Making

The ventral intermediate nucleus (VIM) is the preferred surgical target for treatment of essential tremor. Interventional modalities broadly fall into the categories of lesioning and neuromodulation.

Lesioning of the VIM

Intracranial target lesioning has been completed via a number of strategies. The most widely used lesioning approach is radio-frequency (RF) ablation, which is performed with a tabletop RF lesion generator (Cosman Medical, Burlington, MA). Stereotactic lesioning is completed with the patient awake in the operating room after microelectrode recordings (MERs) or test stimulation prior to ablation. Gamma knife radiation serves as a second option for lesioning the VIM under image-based targeting.[1,2] Appropriate collimation and use of beam-blocking methodologies minimize exposure of the internal capsule. The newest approach approved by the Food and Drug Administration[3] (FDA) is high-intensity focused ultrasound (HIFU; Insightec, Tirat Carmel, Israel) energy aided by direct imaging-based targeting and near real-time magnetic resonance (MR) thermometry in a dedicated interventional magnetic resonance imaging (MRI) suite. Following a complete head shave and placement in a stereotactic head frame, test sonication is completed. In the absence of deficit with test sonication, ablative sonications are completed. No incision is required.

DBS of the VIM

Deep brain stimulation was approved by the FDA in 1997 for the treatment of essential tremor.[4] While it was approved for unilateral implant, bilateral implantation is often completed. In comparison to the lesioning alternatives described previously, neurostimulation as a treatment modality holds the advantages of being reversible, used to treat bilateral symptoms, and amenable to titration. DBS can be completed while awake in the operating room using MER-based targeting or through an approach under anesthesia in which image-based targeting is utilized.[5]

Questions

1. What primary advantages do neurostimulation-based approaches hold over lesioning approaches for the treatment of essential tremor?
2. What factors favor "awake" versus "asleep" DBS completion?

Surgical Procedure

The procedure for DBS electrode placement into the VIM is described. As there are a number of stereotactic systems available, we speak in broad terms regarding the details of the surgical procedure itself. RF lesion generation at the VIM utilizes an identical targeting methodology. Procedural description of HIFU[6] and gamma knife radiosurgery (GKR)[1,2] is beyond the scope of this chapter and has been put forth elsewhere.

Initial trajectory planning is completed in an extraoperative setting utilizing MRI enhanced with gadolinium contrast to assist in avoidance of vasculature. A trajectory that avoids vessels, sulci, and the ventricular system is carefully selected. Because the VIM is not clearly visible on clinical MRI scans, targeting is based on consensus coordinates derived from a Cartesian coordinate system. The midcommissural point (MCP), representing the midpoint between the anterior commissural (AC) point and posterior commissural (PC) point, represents the origin of this coordinate system.

In a mediolateral x-plane, the target coordinate is typically 14–15 mm lateral to the MCP or approximately 11–12 mm lateral to the ventricular wall. Given the somatotopic representation of the VIM, with the upper extremity represented medially, lead placement may be biased 1–2 mm medially with a predominance of upper extremity symptoms and 1–2 mm laterally if lower extremity symptoms are prominent. In an anterior-posterior y-plane, the VIM is 25%–33% of the AC-PC distance posterior to the MCP according to Guiot's geometric scheme.[7] The target in this plane is typically selected 1 mm anterior to the posterior border of the VIM. Finally, in the z-plane, the target is approximately 1 mm deep to the AC-PC plane. While posterior placement of the electrode into the ventral caudalis (Vc) nuclei may result in sensory symptoms, this serves as a useful landmark during awake intraoperative mapping.

Figure 1.1 provides a graphical representation of the VIM consensus coordinates and the relationship between the thalamus and internal capsule at the level of the target. Coronal (Figure 1.1A), parasagittal (Figure 1.1B), and axial (Figure 1.1C) views are shown centered on the VIM target. Figure 1.1D demonstrates a posterior and medial trajectory; the relationship between the trajectory and intracranial nuclei is emphasized. Of note, an ideal trajectory retains an extraventricular pathway that also fails to transgress any pial sulcal boundaries.

Prior to surgery, a thin-cut computed tomographic (CT) scan with a stereotactic frame or skull fiducials may be required in order to transfer the preoperative trajectories to the appropriate stereotactic space. In the operating room, the patient is positioned in a supine or semisitting position. After the head has been prepared and draped in a standard surgical fashion, the selected stereotactic system is used to determine the appropriate entry point for the trajectory. The skin is infiltrated with local anesthetic and an incision centered over the entry point is made. A burr hole is then drilled, after which the dura and pia are opened sharply.

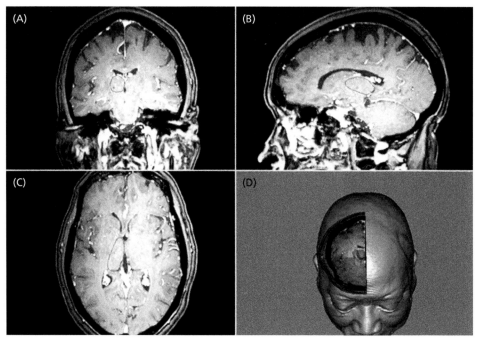

Figure 1.1 VIM targeting. The VIM target is demonstrated in orthogonal views. The thalamus is outlined in pink and the internal capsule in teal. The relationship between these two structures is highlighted. (A) Coronal; (B) parasagittal; (C) axial; and (D) three-dimensional (3D) cutout views are shown. This highlights the 3D relationship between the thalamus and internal capsule. Note that the trajectory is passing in a posterior and medial direction toward the target.

With the stereotacic system defining the predetermined trajectory, intraoperative mapping can begin in the case of awake implantation, or electrode implantation may be immediately performed in the case of implantation under anesthesia. In the former scenario, a microdrive is typically used to allow for fine adjustments of electrode position. MERs may also be performed, which would allow the surgeon to identify tremor cells and cells responsive to passive movement of the patient's extremities. Macrostimulation is typically performed and allows for mapping of the VIM/Vc border as well as evaluation of tremor response. If sensory symptoms are elicited, the electrode is likely within the Vc and as such should be moved 2 mm anteriorly within the Ben-Gun.

Once again, lead placement may be biased 1–2 mm medially with a predominance of upper extremity symptoms and 1–2 mm laterally if lower extremity symptoms are prominent. It is important to note that given the orientation of the thalamus, if an anterior adjustment is made, a concurrent medial adjustment should be considered in order to avoid lateral placement of the electrode. Specifically, for every 2-mm anterior adjustment in the y-axis, a 1-mm medial adjustment in the x-axis should be considered.

In an awake DBS procedure, the final target is customized based on intraoperative MER data and stimulation through the DBS electrode. Two-dimensional imaging data with intraoperative fluoroscopy can help to confirm targeting in the y-axis and the z-axis. In an asleep DBS case, intraprocedural imaging (e.g., MRI, CT) are used to assess lead location relative to the intended trajectory. After the electrode has been implanted in its final position, with the lead secured at the skull surface, the intracranial lead is connected to an extension and tunneled to an internal pulse generator site. This phase II procedure is completed either at the same time or in a delayed fashion.

Oral Boards Review—Management Pearls

1. Generic VIM consensus coordinates in relation to midcommissural point:

VIM Consensus Coordinates	
X	11 mm lateral to the ventricular wall (14–15 mm lateral to the MCP)
Y	25% of AC-PC distance posterior to the MCP
Z	1 mm below the AC-PC plane

2. Considerations for lesioning versus neuromodulation:
   a. Given the reversible nature and potential for therapy titration, neuromodulation is often considered the first-line surgical therapy.
   b. Lesioning often is considered for patients who prefer not to have indwelling hardware, have had a prior infection with indwelling hardware, or have questionable ability to maintain follow-up for therapy titration.
   c. Bilateral neuromodulation can be completed when necessary as bilateral thalamotomies should not be performed.
3. Slightly more lateral targeting in the VIM preferentially treats lower extremity symptoms, whereas more medial targeting treats upper extremity symptoms. Immediately posterior to the VIM is the Vc, and detection of sensory symptoms during intraoperative physiologic mapping defines the posterior border of the VIM.

4. Given the orientation of the thalamus, for every 2-mm anterior adjustment in the *y*-axis one makes intraoperatively, a 1-mm medial adjustment in the *x*-axis should be considered.

Pivot Points

- If a patient has had prior DBS with good effect and has had hardware explantation for treatment of an infection and after treatment of the infection wishes to seek further treatment but does not want hardware reimplanted, then the patient should be considered for a unilateral thalamotomy.
- If a patient has had a prior unilateral thalamotomy for treatment of essential tremor and is now developing worsening symptoms from the nontreated side, then the patient should be considered for neurostimulation-based treatment as opposed to a contralateral thalamotomy.

Aftercare

Postoperative Hospital Course

Following surgery, patients who undergo DBS placement typically undergo a postoperative head CT or MRI to check electrode placement and to assess for any intracranial surgical complications. Patients are observed overnight in either a neurological intensive care unit or a neurological step-down unit. Patients are typically discharged on their preoperative medications on postoperative day 1.

Postoperative Course After Discharge

General practice at most centers involves giving patients intraoperative intravenous antibiotics as well as postoperative oral antibiotics for up to 1 week following surgery.[8] As with most surgeries, patients are instructed to avoid excessive bending, lifting, or twisting for the initial 4–6 weeks after surgery. Patients are encouraged to walk as much as tolerated. They can gently stretch their neck from side to side but are cautioned to avoid quick repetitive neck movements as well as excessive lateral rotation as these maneuvers could cause disruption of the wires. Patients are instructed not to drive until cleared by their surgeon. Patients are warned they may experience soreness in the head, neck, or chest for the first few weeks following surgery. They are often discharged from the hospital with a prescription for a pain medicine. Patients are instructed to notify their surgeon for any flu-like symptoms (e.g., fever above 101.5°F, body aches, chills); severe headaches; increase in redness; swelling; tenderness; drainage from any of the incision sites; numbness; tingling; or changes in sensation of the arms or legs, weakness of the arms or legs, or sudden loss of bowel or bladder control.

Follow-up

If the implanted pulse generator (IPG) and lead extensions are not placed as part of the initial procedure, the patient will be instructed to return between 1 and 2 weeks postoperatively for anterior chest wall IPG implantation as stage II of the DBS implantation procedure. The device is usually kept off until the patient follows up with their movement disorder neurologist for their first postoperative programming session. Patients should follow up with their neurosurgeon 10–14 days following surgery for an incision check. While timing varies from center to center, in the majority of cases, patients will follow up with their movement disorder neurologist for initial programming 1–4 weeks following surgery. The rationale for waiting at least a few weeks following surgery for initial DBS programming is to allow sufficient time for tissue healing and for the microlesional effect to dissipate. The microlesional effect duration can vary from patient to patient. It can last for up to several months but usually starts to fade after the first few weeks when present.[9]

DBS Programming

As with DBS programming in general, each contact is initially tested in monopolar mode to identify the most effective contact. Programming continues in a systematic manner that helps identify the contact pairing and settings that produce the best symptom relief with the fewest side effects. For initial programming, the pulse width and frequency are typically held constant while the voltage is tested at each contact. Once the best contact has been identified, voltage and frequency are adjusted to the lowest levels needed to achieve tremor control without inducing side effects. While there is variability among centers in terms of choice of initial pulse width and voltage settings, we generally start with a low pulse width (60 μs) and a low frequency (130 Hz) in order to allow for increases in these settings in the future if/when they are needed. Some patients, however, do require a higher initial frequency of 160–185 Hz to achieve tremor control.

Given ongoing changes occurring at the electrode-tissue interface, patients often require frequent DBS programming visits in the initial months following surgery in order to fine-tune their settings. Reasons for adjusting a patient's DBS settings include inadequate tremor control, in which case the voltage or frequency may need to be increased or a better contact may need to be identified. The patient may benefit from switching to bipolar or interleaved settings if there is inadequate tremor control with monopolar settings. Another reason for adjusting a patient's DBS settings is if the patient is experiencing side effects such as speech side effects, such as dysarthria or decreased verbal fluency, dysesthesias, dystonia, or disequilibrium. If any of these side effects develops, a different contact(s) likely needs to be chosen or stimulation parameters may need to be reduced. Once DBS settings have been optimized, however, programming visits for the VIM target are usually only necessary biannually or even annually. Typically, patients are instructed to turn their DBS system off while sleeping to conserve battery longevity.

While monopolar stimulation is the most commonly utilized mode for current delivery, bipolar mode is another option if a smaller volume of tissue activation is required. On the other end of the spectrum is the use of double-monopolar stimulation. In this mode, two contacts are used to deliver current, which in turn results in a larger volume of tissue activation, which may be necessary to provide better symptom relief.[8] A large 2016 study looking at battery longevity for 339 batteries in 200 patients with either Parkinson disease or essential tremor observed that bipolar stimulation "was associated with greater longevity than monopolar stimulation (56.1 $\pm$ 3.4 vs. 44.2 $\pm$ 2.1 months; p = 0.006). This effect was most pronounced when stimulation parameters were at low-to-moderate intensity settings. As one would expect, double monopolar configuration was associated with shorter pulse generator longevity than conventional stimulation modes (37.8 $\pm$ 5.6 vs 49.7 $\pm$ 1.9; p = 0.014)."[10] When the IPG has reached its end of service, the patient will typically undergo an outpatient procedure to change the anterior chest wall implant.

Complications and Management

A few large-scale review studies have focused on the complications of DBS surgery. According to a 2005 American Academy of Neurology (AAN) practice parameter for treatment of essential tremor, 18% of patients (37 patients) who had undergone DBS for essential tremor experienced adverse effects from surgery, with 76% of these cases (28 patients) hardware-related issues such as lead displacement or equipment malfunction.[11] In 2006, the AAN published a practice parameter for treatment of Parkinson disease that looked at various studies of patients who had undergone DBS. Although for a different disease, this review identified a number of complications that are relevant to patients undergoing DBS for essential tremor. The adverse surgical complications within 1 month of surgery in order of frequency included infection (5.6%), hemorrhage (3.1%), confusion/disorientation (2.8%), seizures (1.1%), pulmonary embolus (0.6%), cerebrospinal fluid leak (0.6%), peripheral nerve injury (0.6%), and venous infarction (0.3%). The review demonstrated lead compromise (fracture, migration, or malfunction) in 5% of patients necessitating lead replacement. Extension wires had to be replaced in 4.4% of patients (due to erosion or fracture), and the IPG had to be replaced in 4.2% of patients due to malfunction.[12]

As outlined, infection and hemorrhage are the two most common complications reported in the literature. In two large series of over a thousand patients, 5.7% developed an infection, with the majority occurring within 3 months of surgery.[13,14] *Staphylococcus aureus* infections were the most frequent (36%) and were more likely to have earlier onset, pus formation, and a more aggressive development.[14] Infected hardware necessitates temporary, and in some cases permanent, explantation. Several weeks of broad-spectrum intravenous antibiotics are also standard of care in treatment of DBS infections.

A case series of 214 patients and systematic review of the literature on stereotactic procedures looked to analyze the risk factors for hemorrhage.[15] While patients undergoing DBS implantation under image guidance without MERs suffered from symptomatic hemorrhage in 0.5% cases with no patients suffering permanent deficit, a symptomatic hemorrhage rate of 2.1% with permanent deficit or death in 1.1% was reported for patients undergoing DBS with MER in an awake procedure. Risk factors for hemorrhage were specifically noted to include use of MER, number of MER penetrations, as well as sulcal or ventricular involvement by the trajectory.

Additional VIM-specific side effects can include dysarthria, decreased verbal fluency, dysesthesias, disequilibrium/balance disturbance, and dystonia—all of which are stimulation related and resolved with stimulation adjustment.[16-18] Speech disturbance is the

most common side effect of VIM DBS. In a meta-analysis looking at speech disturbance, 19.4% experienced speech difficulty, which occurred more commonly in those
undergoing left-sided or bilateral implantation.[19] Dysarthria can occur if the lead is
placed too far medially (due to stimulation of thalamic connections to the face region)
or too far laterally (due to spread into the internal capsule). Given the typical lateral-to-
medial trajectory of the DBS electrode, if the dysarthria is due to a lead that is too far
medially, using a higher contact may mitigate this side effect by simultaneously moving
the stimulation more laterally. Similarly, if the dysarthria is due to a lead that is placed
too far laterally, a lower contact may help to minimize this side effect by simultaneously
moving the stimulation more medially.

Dysesthesias can occur if the lead is placed too far posteriorly due to stimulation
spread into the Vc nucleus or the lemniscal fibers. Given the typical anterior-to-posterior
trajectory, using a higher contact may obviate this side effect by simultaneously moving
the stimulation more anteriorly.

Balance issues have been reported in 3%–7.5% of patients after VIM DBS. A higher
incidence of balance difficulty has been observed in patients receiving bilateral VIM DBS
compared to unilateral VIM DBS.[8] There is some evidence in the literature to suggest
that reducing the frequency setting to the lowest effective level to achieve tremor control may reduce disequilibrium.[20] Imbalance in VIM DBS can also be due to a lead that
is placed too inferiomedially, with resulting stimulation of the brachium conjunctivum.
In this scenario, using a higher contact may mitigate this side effect.

Oral Boards Review—Complications Pearls

1. Infection is the most common complication from DBS. It occurs in approximately 5% of cases and necessitates hardware removal and long-term
   antibiotics.
2. Hemorrhage from DBS has been correlated with use of MER, number
   of MER penetrations, as well as sulcal or ventricular involvement by the
   trajectory.
3. Speech disturbance is the most common stimulation-related side effect of
   VIM DBS and occurs when the volume of tissue activation is too medial
   (involving the regions of the thalamus with facial connections) or too lateral
   (involving the internal capsule).
4. Paresthesias can occur if the stimulation is too posterior—involving the Vc
   nucleus of the thalamus.

Evidence and Outcomes

Stimulation of the VIM for the treatment of essential tremor has been demonstrated
in numerous studies to be efficacious in reducing tremor at least in the short term[21–24];
however, there are conflicting reports in the literature regarding the long-term efficacy
of VIM stimulation on tremor control. Many studies have shown significant tremor reduction several years after the procedure,[23–25] but others suggested that tremor worsens
with time after DBS. In a study of 91 patients who had undergone unilateral VIM DBS,

patients experienced a 55% improvement in tremor rating scale (TRS) at 1 year, but this effect diminished to 44% at 4 years and 31% at 9 years.[22] Similarly, in a retrospective single-center study of 45 patients, 73% reported waning benefit during a mean follow-up of 56 months (range 12–152 months).[26]

Aside from reducing tremor, VIM DBS has been shown to provide other long-term benefits, such as improving patients' ability to perform ADL, improving overall emotional well-being, and reducing stigma associated with tremor. Specifically, TRS ADLs have been reported at a 73% improvement at 1 year, 52.25% improvement at 4 years, and 36.9% improvement at 9 years.[22] In general, long-term patient satisfaction rates correspond to tremor control.

In conclusion, while more studies are needed to assess the long-term efficacy of VIM DBS for treatment of essential tremor, there are sufficient data to conclude that the procedure produces significant tremor relief initially, with varying degrees of response after the first few years following the procedure. Aside from reducing tremor, VIM DBS has been shown to improve ADLs and emotional well-being and reduce social stigma. Complications are rare, with the most common complication being infection. There is already some evidence showing that recent advances in surgical techniques (asleep DBS vs. the traditional awake procedure with MERs) can reduce the risk of intracranial hemorrhage.[15] Unilateral VIM DBS also appears to be more favorable than bilateral VIM stimulation given the increased risks of dysarthria and disequilibrium with bilateral VIM stimulation. Emerging treatments for essential tremor such as HIFU may play a much larger role in years to come in the treatment of essential tremor, but as with VIM DBS, longitudinal studies are required to evaluate long-term efficacy.

References and Further Reading

1. Witjas, T., et al., A prospective single-blind study of gamma knife thalamotomy for tremor. *Neurology*, 2015. **85**(18): p. 1562–1568.

2. Kooshkabadi, A., et al., Gamma knife thalamotomy for tremor in the magnetic resonance imaging era. *J Neurosurg*, 2013. **118**(4): p. 713–718.

3. FDA approval letter for HIFU. July 11, 2016. Available from https://www.accessdata.fda.gov/scripts/cdrh/cfdocs/cfPMA/pma.cfm?id=P960009

4. FDA approval: DBS for essential tremor.

5. Chen, T., et al., "Asleep" deep brain stimulation for essential tremor. *J Neurosurg*, 2016. **124**(6): p. 1842–1849.

6. Elias, W.J., et al., A pilot study of focused ultrasound thalamotomy for essential tremor. *N Engl J Med*, 2013. **369**(7): p. 640–648.

7. Guiot, G., et al., [Neurophysiologic control procedures for sterotaxic thalamotomy]. *Neurochirurgie*, 1968. **14**(4): p. 553–566.

8. Deuschl, G., et al., Deep brain stimulation: postoperative issues. *Mov Disord*, 2006. **21**(Suppl 14): p. S219–S237.

9. Groiss, S.J., et al., Deep brain stimulation in Parkinson's disease. *Ther Adv Neurol Disord*, 2009. **2**(6): p. 20–28.

10. Almeida, L., et al., Deep brain stimulation battery longevity: comparison of monopolar versus bipolar stimulation modes. *Mov Disord Clin Pract*, 2016. **3**(4): p. 359–366.

11. Zesiewicz, T.A., et al., Practice parameter: therapies for essential tremor: report of the Quality Standards Subcommittee of the American Academy of Neurology. *Neurology*, 2005. **64**(12): p. 2008–2020.

12. Pahwa, R., et al., Practice parameter: treatment of Parkinson disease with motor fluctuations and dyskinesia (an evidence-based review): report of the Quality Standards Subcommittee of the American Academy of Neurology. *Neurology*, 2006. **66**(7): p. 983–995.

13. Tolleson, C., et al., The factors involved in deep brain stimulation infection: a large case series. *Stereotact Funct Neurosurg*, 2014. **92**(4): p. 227–233.

14. Bjerknes, S., et al., Surgical site infections after deep brain stimulation surgery: frequency, characteristics and management in a 10-year period. *PLoS One*, 2014. **9**(8): p. e105288.

15. Zrinzo, L., et al., Reducing hemorrhagic complications in functional neurosurgery: a large case series and systematic literature review. *J Neurosurg*, 2012. **116**(1): p. 84–94.

16. Guzzi, G., et al., Critical reappraisal of DBS targeting for movement disorders. *J Neurosurg Sci*, 2016. **60**(2): p. 181–188.

17. Limousin, P., et al., Multicentre European study of thalamic stimulation in Parkinsonian and essential tremor. *J Neurol Neurosurg Psychiatry*, 1999. **66**(3): p. 289–296.

18. Schuurman, P.R., et al., A comparison of continuous thalamic stimulation and thalamotomy for suppression of severe tremor. *N Engl J Med*, 2000. **342**(7): p. 461–468.

19. Alomar, S., et al., Speech and language adverse effects after thalamotomy and deep brain stimulation in patients with movement disorders: a meta-analysis. *Mov Disord*, 2017. **32**(1): p. 53–63.

20. Ramirez-Zamora, A., H. Boggs, and J.G. Pilitsis, Reduction in DBS frequency improves balance difficulties after thalamic DBS for essential tremor. *J Neurol Sci*, 2016. **367**: p. 122–127.

21. Blomstedt, P., et al., Thalamic deep brain stimulation in the treatment of essential tremor: a long-term follow-up. *Br J Neurosurg*, 2007. **21**(5): p. 504–509.

22. Nazzaro, J.M., R. Pahwa, and K.E. Lyons, Long-term benefits in quality of life after unilateral thalamic deep brain stimulation for essential tremor. *J Neurosurg*, 2012. **117**(1): p. 156–161.

23. Pahwa, R., et al., Long-term evaluation of deep brain stimulation of the thalamus. *J Neurosurg*, 2006. **104**(4): p. 506–512.

24. Rehncrona, S., et al., Long-term efficacy of thalamic deep brain stimulation for tremor: double-blind assessments. *Mov Disord*, 2003. **18**(2): p. 163–170.

25. Sydow, O., et al., Multicentre European study of thalamic stimulation in essential tremor: a six year follow up. *J Neurol Neurosurg Psychiatry*, 2003. **74**(10): p. 1387–1391.

26. Shih, L.C., et al., Loss of benefit in VIM thalamic deep brain stimulation (DBS) for essential tremor (ET): how prevalent is it? *Parkinsonism Relat Disord*, 2013. **19**(7): p. 676–679.

Dominant Essential Tremor

Ashwin Viswanathan

2

Case Presentation

A 78-year-old veteran (A.M.) was referred to our care for surgical treatment of his tremor. The patient does not have tremor while at rest, but the tremor emerges when he holds his arm up against gravity and when performing an action. When eating, writing, and drawing, his tremor becomes severe. He has tremor involving his bilateral upper extremities and is right-handed. A.M. is a widower and lives alone in a remote town in Texas. Obtaining transportation for medical care is burdensome and expensive. He is interested in improving his quality of life through increasing his ability to feed himself, draw, and perform activities of daily living. A.M. requests advice regarding surgical treatment options for his tremor.

Questions

1. How is essential tremor differentiated from Parkinson tremor?
2. What are the surgical options for improving tremor?
3. Which interventions confer an immediate benefit to the patient?

Assessment and Planning

A.M. presents with no resting tremor, but he has kinetic and postural tremor. This is characteristic of essential tremor and distinct from the tremor associated with Parkinson disease, which involves a resting tremor. A.M. has no rigidity or bradykinesia, further supporting the diagnosis of essential tremor.

Surgical interventions for essential tremor include deep brain stimulation (DBS), radio-frequency thalamotomy, laser interstitial thermal therapy (LITT), radiosurgery, and most recently focused ultrasound. DBS has become the most common therapy for essential tremor. As a nonlesional approach, it can be performed bilaterally and hence can treat tremor on both sides of the body. The target for DBS for essential tremor is the ventralis intermedius nucleus (VIM) of the thalamus. In contrast, thalamotomy is typically only performed on one side of the body due to the high complication rate associated with bilateral thalamic lesions.

Multiple techniques for thalamotomy exist. Radio-frequency thalamotomy is a well-established technique with a large volume of clinical experience. It can be performed rapidly and confers an immediate clinical benefit to the patient. More recently, reports exist of thalamotomy performed using LITT. This technique also provides an immediate benefit to the patient and the potential advantage of near real-time monitoring of the lesion using magnetic resonance (MR) thermometry. However, as this procedure is performed with the patient under general anesthesia, it is not possible to monitor the patient for complications during LITT thalamotomy.

Radiosurgery is another well-established technique with a large body of clinical experience. Advantages of radiosurgery include the ability to perform the procedure in patients for whom anticoagulation cannot be stopped. However, there is a delayed treatment effect, with clinical benefit manifesting after 6 months to 1 year.

Most recently, focused ultrasound has emerged as another technique for performing thalamotomy. The advantages of focused ultrasound include an immediate benefit conferred to the patient and the ability to monitor the lesion in near real time. The downside of this technique is the very high startup cost, at least at this time.

Questions

1. What is one disadvantage of radiosurgical thalamotomy?
2. What is the principal advantage of DBS over thalamotomy in the treatment of essential tremor?
3. Name four techniques for performing a thalamotomy.

Oral Boards Review—Diagnostic Pearls

1. For patients who desire bilateral improvement in tremor, DBS is a superior and safer than ablation of the Vim.
2. Radiosurgery and focused ultrasound are techniques that can be offered to patients who cannot stop anticoagulation.
3. The presence of resting tremor, rigidity, or bradykinesia should raise suspicion of Parkinson disease and warrants further clinical workup

---

Decision-Making

Both DBS and thalamotomy are appropriate for this patient to consider. As he has bilateral tremor, DBS affords an opportunity to maximally treat his symptoms. However, after discussion of the need to return monthly for programming and the need for future surgery to change the pulse generator, the patient indicates that he would like a one-time treatment that does not require extensive follow-up.

The various options for thalamotomy are discussed with the patient as well, focusing on the two most common techniques for thalamotomy: radio-frequency and radiosurgical thalamotomy. As radio-frequency thalamotomy confers an immediate benefit to the patient and we have the ability to monitor for complications during the procedure, the patient elects for radio-frequency thalamotomy.

Surgical Procedure

Prior to the procedure, anticoagulants are stopped, and laboratory tests are performed to ensure normal coagulation. Preoperative magnetic resonance imaging (MRI) can aid in targeting the VIM. However, for patients in whom an MRI cannot be performed, preoperative computed tomography (CT) performed with 2-mm cuts can be used to identify the anterior and commissure for indirect targeting.

Frame-based stereotaxy is the most common method for performing radio-frequency thalamotomy. The patient is brought to the operating room. From an anesthetic perspective, benzodiazepines are avoided to allow proper intraoperative evaluation of tremor. A small amount of intravenous propofol and opioids can be used along with the local anesthetic during frame placement.

The CT indicator box is then placed on the frame, and stereotactic CT is performed. This is merged to the preoperative MRI (or preoperative CT) using the stereotactic planning software. The anterior commissure (AC), posterior commissure (PC), and midline plane are chosen on the preoperative image, and the target for the thalamotomy is selected.

The target for the thalamotomy is similar to the standard DBS targeting of the VIM. The target is at the level of the AC-PC plane. A point 10 to 11 mm lateral to the wall of the third ventricle is chosen contralateral to the patient's symptoms. The anterior-posterior location of the target is modified to be between 21% and 25% of the AC-PC distance anterior to the posterior commissure.

The goal of thalamotomy is the creation of an approximately 6-mm lesion in the superior inferior plane. To accomplish this, a radio-frequency electrode with 2mm of exposed tip can be used. The tip diameter can be the surgeon's preference; however, a tip diameter of 1.2 mm allows the radio-frequency probe to fit within the standard cannulas used for DBS. Figure 2.1 details the intraoperative setup and equipment needed for radio-frequency thalamotomy.

The patient is prepared and draped, and an intraoperative imager such as a fluoroscope or intraoperative CT is positioned. Minimal shaving is needed. The side of the patient's tremor and the side of the intended thalamotomy are triple checked along with the frame coordinates. A standard entry point of 12 cm behind the nasion and 3 cm lateral to midline is chosen. The entry point is chosen to be lateral enough to avoid a transventricular trajectory. The procedure can be performed either through a twist-drill entry or through a burr hole. I chose a burr hole to permit visualization of the cortical entry point and to permit intraoperative movement of the radio-frequency electrode if needed.

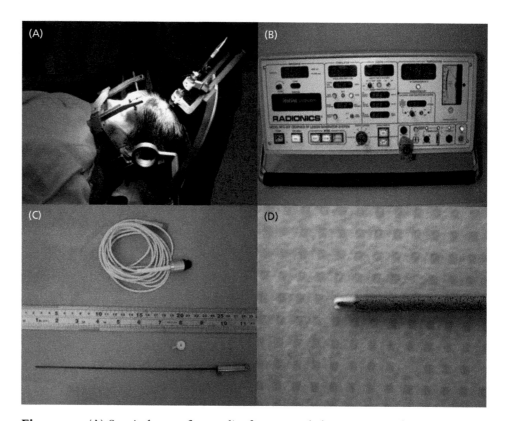

Figure 2.1 (A) Surgical setup for a radio-frequency thalamotomy can be minimalistic. A minimal shave and draping are adequate for performing the procedure. (B) The Radionics radio-frequency generator has historically been used for the procedure. This generator has been updated by Cosman Medical and now Boston Scientific. (C) A 1.2-mm radio-frequency probe with a 2-mm exposed tip is a safe choice for both radio-frequency thalamotomy and pallidotomy. (D) An enlarged view of the tip of the radio-frequency electrode. Images courtesy of Dr. Kim Burchiel.

The radio-frequency electrode is deployed to the target, and intraoperative testing is performed. It is essential to document the amplitude and characteristic of the patient's tremor prior to insertion of the radio-frequency electrode to be able to recognize a lesional effect from the insertion of the radio-frequency probe. High-frequency stimulation using 50 Hz is performed to ensure a sensory threshold greater than 0.5 V. Low-frequency stimulation at 2 Hz is performed to ensure a motor threshold greater than 1 V. Should the patient not reach this criterion, the electrode is repositioned either anteriorly (sensory) or medially (motor), and testing is repeated. Intraoperative imaging can help determine if a stereotactic error exists.

Finally, stimulation at 180 Hz is used to ensure tremor suppression at low levels (0.1–0.5 V). Once this is confirmed, three lesions are performed at the target, +2 mm, and –2 mm at 70°C for 60 seconds. The radio-frequency probe is removed, and a miniplate is placed over the burr hole prior to closing.

Oral Boards Review—Management Pearls

1. Bilateral thalamotomy is a high-risk intervention and should be avoided.
2. The use of intraoperative imaging such as CT can minimize the risk of the procedure by confirming the position of the radio-frequency electrode prior to lesion creation.
3. It is essential to perform radio-frequency thalamotomy in the awake, cooperative patient to permit intraoperative testing, with the goal of minimizing complications.

Pivot Points

1. Intraoperative capsular side effects at an amplitude less than 1 V warrant repositioning of the radio-frequency electrode more medially. An intraoperative CT scan can guide repositioning of the electrode.
2. Should the patient's tremor contralateral to the treated arm become bothersome, DBS should be offered, as opposed to contralateral thalamotomy.
3. In the event of symptom recurrence in the treated arm, repeat thalamotomy can be performed using an identical surgical technique but with increasing the lesion temperature to 72°C.

Aftercare

Postoperatively, the patient is admitted for observation. A careful neurological exam is performed to assess for neurological deficit and sensory disturbance after thalamotomy. The patient is mobilized as soon as feasible, with no period of bed rest. A routine postoperative CT to assess for intracranial bleeding is good practice. An MRI with contrast to delineate the thalamotomy can be performed at the 3-month time window.

Complications and Management

The risks of radio-frequency thalamotomy include contralateral weakness (10%–15%) and dysarthria (5%). However, most series reporting complications of radio-frequency thalamotomy were prior to the common use of three-dimensional intraoperative imaging.

Radiosurgical thalamotomy is a safe procedure, and complications can be dose related. Risks of this procedure include persistent symptoms (15%–20%), motor impairment (5%), and speech impairment (3%).

Focused ultrasound is a newer technique for performing thalamotomy. However, in initial experiences, there may be a 30%–40% risk of gait disturbance in the immediate postoperative period, which reduces to 10%–15% of patients with persistent complications at 1 year.

Oral Boards Review—Complications Pearls

1. Frequent intraoperative CT scanning during spinal needle advancement can prevent unintentional insertion of the spinal needle into the spinal cord.
2. Motor weakness can usually be avoided by ensuring that a motor threshold of 1 V is achieved during intraoperative stimulation.
3. Two lesions are recommended to avoid the risk of underlesioning the spinothalamic tract.

Evidence and Outcomes

Radio-frequency thalamotomy is an effective procedure for essential tremor. Between 60% and 80% of patients will maintain excellent improvement, with either no tremor or significant improvement in tremor. Repeat radio-frequency thalamotomy has also been shown to be effective and can be performed using a temperature of 72°C.

Radiosurgery has similarly been shown to be an effective strategy for treating tremor. A recent large retrospective series demonstrated that when using a median dose of 140 Gy, 60% of patients experienced tremor arrest or a barely perceptible tremor (Niranjan et al. 2017). Of those patients who did have tremor improvement, 96% of patients maintained the benefit in the longer term.

Clinical experience with focused ultrasound thalamotomy continues to increase. In a randomized, sham-controlled study, patients assigned to thalamotomy experienced a 40% reduction in tremor scores as compared with a 0.1% improvement in tremor scores in patients who underwent a sham procedure (Elias et al. 2016).

References and Further Reading

Akbostanci MC, Slavin KV, Burchiel KJ. Stereotactic ventral intermedial thalamotomy for the treatment of essential tremor: results of a series of 37 patients. *Stereotact Funct Neurosurg.* 1999;72(2–4):174–177.

Elias WJ, Lipsman N, Ondo WG, Ghanouni P, Kim YG, Lee W, Schwartz M, Hynynen K, Lozano AM, Shah BB, Huss D, Dallapiazza RF, Gwinn R, Witt J, Ro S, Eisenberg HM, Fishman PS, Gandhi D, Halpern CH, Chuang R, Butts Pauly K, Tierney TS, Hayes MT, Cosgrove GR, Yamaguchi T, Abe K, Taira T, Chang JW. A randomized trial of focused ultrasound thalamotomy for essential tremor. *N Engl J Med.* 2016 Aug 25;375(8):730–739.

Harris M, Steele J, Williams R, Pinkston J, Zweig R, Wilden JA. MRI-guided laser interstitial thermal thalamotomy for medically intractable tremor disorders. *Mov Disord.* 2019 Jan;34(1):124–129.

Kooshkabadi A, Lunsford LD, Tonetti D, Flickinger JC, Kondziolka D. Gamma knife thalamotomy for tremor in the magnetic resonance imaging era. *J Neurosurg.* 2013 Apr;118(4):713–718.

Niranjan A, Raju SS, Kooshkabadi A, Monaco E 3rd, Flickinger JC, Lunsford LD. Stereotactic radiosurgery for essential tremor: retrospective analysis of a 19-year experience. *Mov Disord.* 2017 May;32(5):769–777.

Ohye C, Higuchi Y, Shibazaki T, Hashimoto T, Koyama T, Hirai T, Matsuda S, Serizawa T, IIori T, IIayashi M, Ochiai T, Samura H, Yamashiro K. Gamma knife thalamotomy for Parkinson disease and essential tremor: a prospective multicenter study. Neurosurgery. 2012 Mar;70(3):526–535; discussion 535–536.

Non–Tremor-Predominant Parkinson Disease

Thomas Ostergard and Jonathan P. Miller

3

Case Presentation

A 44-year-old woman presents with a 6-year history of abnormal movements. Her symptoms initially began with a mild resting tremor in the left hand, which then progressed to involve the right hand. Over time, she developed disabling episodes of bradykinesia and freezing, both predominantly involving the upper extremities. She was initially prescribed ropinirole but was without improvement in her symptoms. Levodopa resulted in a dramatic and sustained improvement in her symptoms. However, she requires a progressively increased dosage of medication for relief of bradykinesia, and this is associated with worsening dyskinetic movements that start shortly after each levodopa dose. Her current medication regimen also includes amantadine and rasagiline.

Her greatest complaint is the bradykinesia when off medication, which produces difficulty typing, writing, and cooking. Her second most limiting symptom is the medication-induced dyskinesia and the resulting fluctuations between too much and too little movement. She has no complaints regarding falls and denies any symptoms of autonomic dysfunction but does complain of symptoms consistent with restless legs syndrome. On examination (on medication), she has no noticeable tremor. Her gait is slow with stooped posture but without signs of central ataxia. She has moderate dyskinesia. Her examination is otherwise unremarkable. No cerebellar signs are present on examination, and she denies any bulbar or respiratory complaints.

Questions

1. What is the most likely diagnosis?
2. What conditions can mimic these symptoms?
3. What are the next steps in management?

Assessment and Planning

The patient undergoes volumetric magnetic resonance imaging (MRI) with double-dose gadolinium to rule out other disorders as well as assist with possible preoperative planning; the imaging shows no abnormalities. She also undergoes examination on and off levodopa to assess responsiveness to that medication. Her Unified Parkinson Disease Rating Scale Part III (UPDRS-III) off medication is 31, which improves to 12.5 on medication. Her neuropsychiatric testing reveals some subcortical processing inefficiency consistent with the diagnosis of Parkinson disease (PD) but otherwise no abnormalities. This patient appears to have significant functional impairment from motor fluctuations, including levodopa-responsive nontremor symptoms of PD and side effects of treatment. Her case is discussed in a multidisciplinary conference, and she is deemed to be a good candidate for deep brain stimulation (DBS; bilateral subthalamic nucleus [STN]) to improve these symptoms.

The main motor symptoms of PD are a 4- to 6-Hz tremor, bradykinesia, and rigidity. Other common motor findings consist of loss of postural reflex, flexed posture, and freezing. Tremor is commonly the most clinically obvious symptom. However, because it is a resting tremor and therefore improves with action, it is usually not as functionally limiting as the nontremor symptoms of PD. Bradykinesia is common and often the most functionally limiting. Other common nontremor symptoms of PD include soft voice, micrographia, ataxia, sleep disorders, and a variety of mood (frequently depression) and cognitive disorders.

Parkinson disease can be roughly categorized into tremor-dominant PD and postural instability and gait difficulty (PIGD) PD. Patients with tremor-dominant PD appear to have a slower progression, with a lower mean age at onset and a poorer response to levodopa. The PIGD subtype is associated with more rapid progression of cognitive decline with a higher rate of dementia. Because of this finding, when discussing patients with a PIGD subtype, it is important to include detailed neuropsychiatric evaluation during the preoperative workup because there are important implications for candidacy and target selection.

While there is often consensus between members of the multidisciplinary team, neurosurgeons must remain skeptical when a patient carries a diagnosis of PD. Postmortem studies have shown that a clinical diagnosis of PD is correct in only 75%–95% of cases, which is extremely important to remember when considering a preponderance of nontremor symptoms. Common mimickers of idiopathic PD include multiple system atrophy (MSA), progressive supranuclear palsy (PSP), diffuse Lewy body disease, corticobasal ganglionic degeneration, vascular Parkinsonism, normal-pressure hydrocephalus, and drug-induced Parkinsonism. The majority of these disorders have clinical features and radiographic findings that clearly differentiate them from PD. The true difficulty lies in differentiating idiopathic PD from either PSP or MSA. There can be significant difficulty in differentiating these three disease processes due to a high frequency of atypical presentation and symptom overlap. This chapter therefore only briefly focuses on the common and most obvious differences to assist in clinical diagnosis.

Progressive supranuclear palsy is the most common neurodegenerative disease that mimics idiopathic PD. Patients with PSP have an early onset of ataxia and often complain of falls. Ataxia in idiopathic PD is frequently seen much later in the disease and is a less common complaint in patients with PD. Patients with PSP also frequently have more prominent cognitive issues, including cognitive slowing, personality changes, and social withdrawal.

Multiple system atrophy is classified into three subgroups, depending on which system produces the greatest symptoms. The striatonigral degeneration subset has predominant extrapyramidal symptoms and is therefore the most likely to be confused with idiopathic PD. In contrast to idiopathic PD, tremor in MSA is usually symmetric at onset and shows a poorer response to treatment with levodopa. Other clues that should raise suspicion of MSA include multiple autonomic symptoms, early-onset ataxia, and significant dystonia.

It is important to screen patients' medications to rule out drug-induced Parkinsonism. Common medications that can cause Parkinsonism include dopamine release inhibitors such as typical and atypical antipsychotics, drugs that deplete dopamine stores (reserpine), and dopamine antagonists (lithium, tricyclic antidepressants).

Due to referral patterns, neurosurgeons are unlikely to frequently encounter many of these conditions. The Movement Disorder Society has created a set of diagnostic criteria that are helpful when approaching this lack of exposure. The diagnosis of PD should be questioned whenever "red flags" are present. The easiest of these to clinically diagnose are rapid progression to immobility, absent progression of symptoms, early bulbar dysfunction, inspiratory respiratory dysfunction, early severe autonomic dysfunction (within the first 5 years of disease), and bilateral symmetric symptoms.

These features, along with neuroimaging findings, should be discussed with the multidisciplinary team to confirm a diagnosis of idiopathic PD. The patient should then be counseled about the risks and benefits of DBS implantation. When discussing potential benefits, it should be emphasized that only dopamine-responsive (nontremor) symptoms are likely to improve. To properly manage expectations, patients should also be counseled that their symptoms are unlikely to improve more than "on periods."

If they have not already done so, candidates for DBS implantation should be evaluated by a movement disorder neurologist prior to consideration. This provides an opportunity to confirm the clinical diagnosis as well as confirm that all appropriate pharmacologic therapies have been attempted. On confirmation of the clinical diagnosis, the neurosurgeon should assess the patient's overall health status to better determine the risks and benefits of surgery. The patient is then evaluated by a neuropsychologist to exclude the presence of psychiatric conditions or dementia. These data are compiled and discussed at a multidisciplinary conference to determine which patients should undergo implantation. Patients then undergo MRI to assist with preoperative planning as well as exclude other causes of PD.

Oral Boards Review—Diagnostic Pearls

1. In patients with non–tremor-predominant symptoms, a multidisciplinary evaluation is key to determine potential surgical candidates.
2. Nontremor manifestations of PD include bradykinesia; rigidity; soft voice; micrographia; shuffling steps; ataxia; sleep apnea and sleep disorders; changes in mood (depression, anxiety, apathy); and cognition (memory difficulties, dementia).
3. It is important to differentiate medication side effects and true symptoms. The choice of STN or globus pallidus internus (GPi) implantation can significantly impact which symptoms improve with stimulation.
4. It is important to differentiate PD mimickers if someone has predominant nontremor symptoms. Most mimickers of PD have little improvement with DBS.

Decision-Making

The choice of stimulation target for the treatment of PD is controversial; however, there is an increasing body of literature to help guide surgeons. There are five large randomized controlled trials (RCTs) with multiple reports regarding their outcome[1–3] and one meta-analysis. Importantly, all five RCTs showed no difference in overall motor outcome. However, some of the secondary outcomes do help guide choice of stimulation target.

Targeting the STN has shown superior improvement in bradykinesia. It has also significantly decreased treatment expense due to lower energy requirement for stimulation, leading to fewer generator changes.[4] This target allows for a significant reduction in levodopa requirement.[1,2] Targeting the STN is less effective for axial-predominant symptoms, such as postural instability and gait freezing. Improvements in gait from STN DBS are mainly due to improvements in stride length and speed due to improvement in bradykinesia. There is also a higher incidence of cognitive decline with STN DBS.

Questions

1. Which target (STN vs. GPi) is more likely to reduce levodopa requirements?
2. Which is the favored target for the cognitively impaired patient with PD who will be undergoing DBS?
3. Which target (STN vs. GPi) will lead to a better overall motor outcome?

The GPi directly targets dyskinesia and is likely more effective at improving dyskinesia.[1] The improvement in dyskinesia due to STN stimulation is thought to be secondary to the significant decrease in levodopa requirement.[5] Stimulation of the GPi has also shown better outcomes for levodopa-responsive gait and balance.

Surgical Procedure

Surgical implantation techniques for DBS leads vary considerably, and there is no consensus on the most effective approach. Classically, electrodes have been implanted using framed stereotaxy, minimal sedation, and microelectrode recording (MER), although excellent results have also been obtained using intraoperative imaging under general anesthesia and frameless stereotaxy. The description that follows is in regard to the use of a framed system as this requires additional consideration in the approach.

For framed stereotaxy, the patient is placed in a stereotactic frame with the base of the frame aligned with a line between the lateral canthus and tragus, roughly approximating the plane between the anterior commissure and posterior commissure. The patient should be centered in the frame without any contact between the patient and the edges of the frame. Depending on the frame system used, various techniques (straps, external auditory canal bars, etc.) are used to stabilize the frame during placement.

Optimal pin placement is important to avoid morbidity and allow for ideal targeting. When placing frontal pins, the key structures to avoid are the frontal sinus, supraorbital nerves, and frontal (also known as the temporal) branches of the facial nerve. The placement of posterior pins is guided by the dural venous sinuses and mastoid air cells.

The pins should be localized to areas that will minimize radiographic scatter into target regions. It should always be remembered that acoustic transmission is much greater through bone, so that any metal contact with the frame (especially by screwdrivers) will be much louder to the patient. The anxiety associated with frame placement usually worsens movement disorder symptoms and occasionally requires mild sedation for frame placement.

Pins should be tightened with enough torque to gain purchase in the outer table of the skull, but not tight enough to cause distortion of the frame or skull fracture. If the patient leaves the operating room area for imaging after frame placement, a member of the surgical team must accompany the patient with tools to remove the frame and knowledge of how to do so. Should an issue arise during transport, most importantly an airway problem, the frame may need to be urgently removed. If intraoperative imaging is available, frame placement can be performed in the operating room.

Volumetric imaging must include the skin of the cranial vertex and the anterior, posterior, and superior portions of the frame. This image is then co-registered and fused to the image from the preoperative MRI, and the target is localized (Figure 3.1). To complete the electrode trajectory, a surface entry point must be selected. The entry point should be at the apex of a cortical gyrus to avoid venous structures that run in the sulci. It is important to avoid the large parasagittal veins that drain into the superior sagittal sinus. A "fly-through" of the trajectory, evaluating it on every axial slice, should be used to confirm that the planned trajectory does not traverse any vascular structures. The lateral ventricles should be avoided, if possible, to reduce the chance of hemorrhage from ependymal vessels as well as to reduce loss of cerebrospinal fluid, which could compromise targeting.

Once planning has been completed, the patient is positioned supine, and light sedation is given to minimize anxiety during initial surgical exposure. An upright position may allow for air entry and shift of intracranial contents, so a supine position is likely to be superior to a sitting position. The anesthesia team is advised regarding the need for antibiotic administration prior to incision, as well as the need to limit spikes in

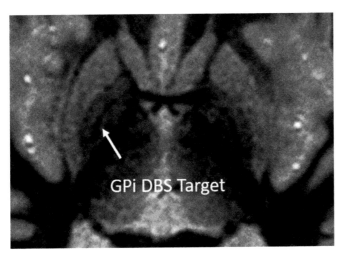

Figure 3.1 Axial inversion recovery weighted MRI sequence delineates the boundaries of the globus pallidus externus versus the globus pallidus internus. The DBS target within the posteroventral globus pallidus internus is marked.

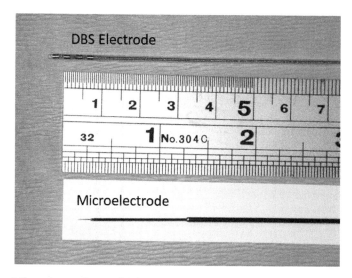

Figure 3.2 Microelectrodes are high-impedance electrodes that allow recording of single-unit activity. Microelectrodes have tip diameters measured in micrometers, as opposed to the diameter of the DBS electrode, which is usually 1.27 mm.

blood pressure, which may increase the risk of hemorrhage during electrode placement. Monitoring devices and intravenous lines should preferentially be placed on the upper extremity with less severe symptoms so that testing is unimpeded on the more severe side. The frame is set to the first trajectory, and a blunt probe is used through the reducing tube to localize the center of the incision. The first target should be contralateral to the patient's worst symptoms. Should the procedure be aborted before the second electrode is placed, the patient's worst symptoms will still be treated. The first trajectory is also less influenced by brain shift due to loss of cerebrospinal fluid, potentially allowing for more accurate targeting. The burr hole is placed, and the dura, arachnoid, and pia are opened.

The electrode is implanted by either MER or stereotactic guidance. If performing MER, the patient's symptoms are tested during stimulation to assess for improvement as well as side effects. When using MER, the combination of anatomical knowledge and the patient's symptoms during stimulation allows the surgeon to know where the electrode has been placed and what, if any, adjustments need to be made (Figure 3.2). Once the lead is in place, intraoperative testing allows for assessment of efficacy (particularly for rigidity) and off-target stimulation side effects. See the Pivot Points for discussion of changes in trajectory. Use of advanced intraoperative imaging may obviate the need for awake mapping and testing, although this is controversial (Figure 3.3).

The lead is anchored in place by either a device or a relief loop secured by suture. If a retention device is used, the outer table of the skull must be contoured to accept the device and minimize the risk of skin erosion over the device. The leads are protected by rubber coverings and tunneled inferolaterally to the ipsilateral side of the planned implantable pulse generator location. Implantation of the pulse generator can be performed immediately afterward or in a delayed fashion.

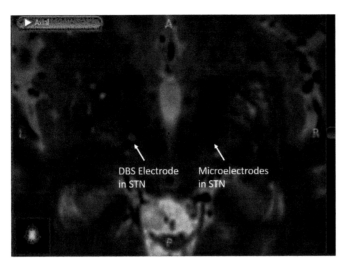

Figure 3.3 Intraoperative CT merged with a preoperatively obtained MRI (axial section) demonstrates the DBS electrode within the left STN and three microelectrodes within the right STN.

Oral Boards Review—Management Pearls

1. Excellent level 1 evidence has shown that DBS treatment is vastly superior to maximal medical therapy.
2. Significant improvement is usually only seen in dopamine-responsive symptoms.
3. The STN is a favorable target in patients with bradykinesia; the GPi is favored for patients with significant dyskinesia or ataxia or cognitive issues.

Oral Boards Review—Pivot Points

1. Stimulation-induced side effects can inform the surgeon about the relative position of the electrode. When targeting the STN, if a patient experiences gaze deviation, dysarthria, or muscle contraction, then the electrode is stimulating the corticospinal tract and therefore is anterolateral to target. Paresthesias are due to stimulation of the medial lemniscus, indicating the electrode is posterior to the target. Diplopia (as opposed to conjugate gaze deviation) is due to oculomotor nerve stimulation from an anteromedially placed electrode.
2. When targeting the GPi, corticospinal tract stimulation is due to placement medial to the target. Photopsia is due to optic tract stimulation from placement anterior and deep (ventral) to the target.

Aftercare

Following implantation, patients are continued on their home movement disorder medications. Postoperative volumetric computed tomography (CT) is performed to evaluate for asymptomatic hemorrhage. This study provides two additional important data points. It allows for reregistration with the preoperative MRI to confirm the accuracy of electrode placement. This feedback is important to allow surgeons to evaluate accuracy. Additionally, if an implanted pulse generator (IPG) is added in a delayed fashion, the scout film from the postoperative CT can be used to estimate the location of the electrode tips, which allows for minimizing the size of the incision as well as inadvertent electrode damage.

If there are no intraoperative complications or evidence of postoperative hemorrhage, patients are monitored overnight and discharged the next morning. Patients with perielectrode hemorrhage are kept in a monitored setting with strict blood pressure control. PGI frequently occurs in a staged manner within a few weeks of surgery but can also be implanted during lead implantation. Patients are seen in clinic for programming several weeks after surgery, at which point the microlesional effect of implantation should have subsided.

Complications and Their Management

The most feared complication following DBS is electrode-associated intracerebral hemorrhage. Large series have shown that the incidence of electrode-associated hemorrhage is roughly 1.5% per electrode.[6] Because most patients undergo bilateral implantation, this translates to a 3% hemorrhage rate per patient. Permanent deficit from electrode-associated hemorrhage occurs in roughly 0.5% of cases.[6] There is likely increased risk in older patients or patients with a history of hypertension. Given the current controversy regarding the use of intraoperative MER, it should be noted that there is a significantly increased risk of electrode-associated hemorrhage with MER.[6,7]

During awake DBS, electrode-associated hemorrhage is usually diagnosed by new clinical symptoms. It should be suspected whenever there is slow loss of MER signals, indicating that the electrode may be inside a hematoma. If fluoroscopy is being used for the procedure, a repeat radiograph can be taken to evaluate if an expanding hematoma has caused electrode displacement. During procedures under general anesthesia, often the only symptom is unexplained systemic hypertension.

On identification of electrode-associated hemorrhage, the procedure should be halted. The electrode is left in place to potentially assist with tamponade. Following recovery, there is also the potential to use the electrode in the future. The frame should be removed, and the patient should immediately have a CT performed. Given the potential for rapid expansion and resultant loss of airway control, a member of the anesthesia team should remain with the patient until the extent of the hemorrhage is identified.

The remainder of management is mainly extrapolated from data regarding the management of spontaneous intracerebral hemorrhage. Blood pressure should be tightly controlled to reduce the risk of expansion. Surgical evacuation of an intracerebral hemorrhage is somewhat controversial; however, some data suggest that, if evacuated, early evacuation is better than late evacuation. If evacuation is pursued, a minimally invasive or endoscopic approach is likely best. When evaluating for the need for hematoma removal or hemicraniectomy, it should be remembered that significant edema will develop around the hematoma within 72 hours.

Surgical site infection occurs in roughly 5%[8] but almost always involves the IPG incision and rarely occurs at the cranial wound. Management of this complication requires removal of the infected hardware and treatment with appropriate antibiotics. For these patients, there will be a period without stimulation while the infection heals, before a new IPG can be implanted. A trial should be performed to evaluate the severity of the patient's symptoms without stimulation. If debilitating, consideration can be given to performance of radio-frequency lesioning using the intracranial electrode.

Whenever there is an unexplained significant change in hemodynamics or oxygenation, the possibility of air embolism should be considered. When routine monitoring is used, the rate of asymptomatic air embolism in the semisitting position has been reported as roughly 20%. However, symptomatic air embolism has been reported to occur in only roughly 1% of DBS cases.[9]

A subset of patients presents with delayed, gradual decompensation following implantation; these patients are found to have significant edema surrounding the length of the electrodes. The pathophysiology of this condition is still unknown. Unless there are other signs of infection, there is no need to undergo extensive investigation for an infectious etiology. As discussed, intracranial infection from DBS is an extremely rare entity. Most surgeons administer steroids, with case reports describing a good response to oral steroids. This condition usually presents in subacute fashion after implantation and resolves in a variable time frame. While this condition is rare, it is important to remember to prevent unnecessary hardware removal.

Poor clinical response to therapy should prompt reassessment of patient and target selection, electrode placement, programming parameters, or hardware malfunction. By coregistering repeat imaging with preoperative imaging, electrode location can be confirmed. Hardware and programming issues should be evident through device interrogation. The patient should be reassessed to confirm the clinical diagnosis of PD. If the electrode is not accurately placed, then even minimal repositioning of the lead appears effective.

If the electrodes are properly positioned and functioning correctly, then they are likely providing some benefit and therefore should not be removed. A "rescue lead" can be implanted into the unimplanted site (GPi or STN) as salvage therapy. Implantation of the STN to "rescue" a poor response to GPi stimulation has shown good efficacy. Similarly, implantation of GPi to rescue a poor response to STN stimulation also appears effective.

Oral Boards Review—Complication Pearls

1. Infection is the most common complication and usually requires explantation of the IPG, but not always the cranial hardware.
2. Intracranial hemorrhage is the most feared complication, occurring in 3% of patients, leaving 0.6% of patients with a permanent deficit.

3. If hemorrhage is suspected, the patient should be closely monitored for airway compromise and immediately taken for CT. Management is largely guided by data from spontaneous Intracranial Hemorrhage (ICH) trials.

4. Noninfectious perielectrode edema is rare but is important to recognize to prevent unnecessary explantation.

5. If there is poor clinical response to stimulation, after troubleshooting, consider a rescue electrode in an alternate target.

Evidence and Outcomes

There is excellent level 1 evidence that DBS works better than medical therapy, with improved motor function[3,10,11] and quality of life.[10] Appropriate patient selection is paramount to achieve optimal patient outcomes. The UPDRS is used to compare clinical outcomes following trials of DBS. Objective motor symptoms are scored by part III and consist of grading of rest tremor, rigidity, speech, posture, and so on. RCTs[3,10-13] have shown roughly 30%–40% improvement in UPDRS-III scores. Most patients experience sustained benefit similar to their best response to medications. Although there is no difference in motor outcome based on target, STN implantation is associated with much greater reduction in levodopa and less need for generator replacement, whereas GPi is associated with better dyskinesia suppression and less labor-intensive programming and medication adjustment.

The UPDRS-II score assesses activities of daily living during "on" and "off" symptoms. When assessed off medication, this metric should highlight the worst of a patient's symptoms. Following DBS, UPDRS-II scores decrease between 10% and 40%. As discussed, STN DBS allows for a significant reduction in dopaminergic medications and significantly decreases dyskinesias. When GPi is targeted, there is no reduction in dopaminergic medications; however, there is direct reduction of dyskinesias.

Deep brain stimulation for PD is one of the best studied surgical procedures in neurosurgery. It can have a significant impact on a patient's function and has been proven to improve quality of life.[10] By careful patient selection, thoughtful planning, and good surgical technique, neurosurgeons have the opportunity to make a significant impact on the lives of patients with PD.

References and Further Reading

1. Burchiel KJ, Anderson VC, Favre J, Hammerstad JP: Comparison of pallidal and subthalamic nucleus deep brain stimulation for advanced Parkinson's disease: results of a randomized, blinded pilot study. *Neurosurgery* 45:1375–1382; discussion 1382–1374, 1999.

2. Follett KA, Weaver FM, Stern M, Hur K, Harris CL, Luo P, et al: Pallidal versus subthalamic deep-brain stimulation for Parkinson's disease. *N Engl J Med* 362:2077–2091, 2010.

3. Weaver FM, Follett K, Stern M, Hur K, Harris C, Marks WJ Jr, et al.: Bilateral deep brain stimulation vs best medical therapy for patients with advanced Parkinson disease: a randomized controlled trial. *JAMA* 301:63–73, 2009.

4. Williams NR, Foote KD, Okun MS: STN vs. GPi deep brain stimulation: translating the re-match into clinical practice. *Mov Disord Clin Pract* 1:24–35, 2014.

5. Deuschl G, Schade-Brittinger C, Agid Y, Group ES: Neurostimulation for Parkinson's disease with early motor complications. *N Engl J Med* 368:2038, 2013.

6. Binder DK, Rau GM, Starr PA: Risk factors for hemorrhage during microelectrode-guided deep brain stimulator implantation for movement disorders. *Neurosurgery* 56: 722–732; discussion 722–732, 2005.

7. Hariz MI: Complications of deep brain stimulation surgery. *Mov Disord* 17(Suppl 3):S162–S166, 2002.

8. Sillay KA, Larson PS, Starr PA: Deep brain stimulator hardware-related infections: incidence and management in a large series. *Neurosurgery* 62:360–366; discussion 366–367, 2008.

9. Chang EF, Cheng JS, Richardson RM, Lee C, Starr PA, Larson PS: Incidence and management of venous air embolisms during awake deep brain stimulation surgery in a large clinical series. *Stereotact Funct Neurosurg* 89:76–82, 2011.

10. Deuschl G, Schade-Brittinger C, Krack P, Volkmann J, Schafer H, Botzel K, et al.: A randomized trial of deep-brain stimulation for Parkinson's disease. *N Engl J Med* 355:896–908, 2006.

11. Schuepbach WM, Rau J, Knudsen K, Volkmann J, Krack P, Timmermann L, et al.: Neurostimulation for Parkinson's disease with early motor complications. *N Engl J Med* 368:610–622, 2013.

12. Williams A, Gill S, Varma T, Jenkinson C, Quinn N, Mitchell R, et al.: Deep brain stimulation plus best medical therapy versus best medical therapy alone for advanced Parkinson's disease (PD SURG trial): a randomised, open-label trial. *Lancet Neurol* 9:581–591, 2010.

13. Witt K, Daniels C, Reiff J, Krack P, Volkmann J, Pinsker MO, et al.: Neuropsychological and psychiatric changes after deep brain stimulation for Parkinson's disease: a randomised, multicentre study. *Lancet Neurol* 7:605–614, 2008.

Tremor-Dominant Parkinson Disease

Stephanie Zyck and Gaddum Duemani Reddy

Case Presentation

A 65-year-old right-handed male is referred with a 10-year history of bilateral upper extremity tremors. The symptoms started in the right arm, but within a couple of years, they began to involve the left arm as well. The tremor is worse at rest but also present with movements. On further history, he reports mild difficulty with initiating movements and overall stiffness that presented approximately 5 years after the tremor. He was initially treated for essential tremor with minimal benefit from propranolol. With the appearance of the additional symptoms, he was diagnosed with Parkinson disease (PD) by his neurologist. He was started on medications, with improvement in the stiffness and initial tremor improvement. Recently, he has required increased dosages to maintain medication efficacy and developed worsened motor fluctuations. He is currently unable to perform his activities of daily living.

Questions

1. What is the likely diagnosis?
2. What are the subtypes of PD, and how are they differentiated?
3. Which tests can be used to differentiate PD from essential tremor?
4. What is the appropriate initial therapy?

Assessment and Planning

Despite the patient having mild symptoms except for tremor, the functional neurosurgeon strongly suspects PD. PD in and of itself is a heterogeneous disorder that can present with differing symptomatology. The most common subclassification separates a tremor-dominant subtype from a non–tremor-dominant subtype, also known as a bradykinetic-rigid subtype or postural instability and gait difficulty (PIGD). This subclassification relies solely on subsections of the Unified Parkinson Disease Rating Scale (UPDRS) or the more recent Movement Disorder Society Unified Parkinson Disease Rating Scale (MDS-UPDRS). A ratio is generated by dividing average scores on the tremor questions by average scores on movement and gait subsections. If this ratio is greater than 1.15, the classification is tremor dominant. If the ratio is less than 0.9, the classification is PIGD. Scores between 0.9 and 1.15 are considered indeterminate.

However, essential tremor also remains on the differential. These two differing movement disorders are classically differentiated based on clinical presentation, but in practice there are several overlapping features that make it difficult to differentiate between them. Further complicating the issue is the possibility that both pathologies can exist in the same patient. Additional noninvasive tests, such as measure of tremor frequency using accelerometry, can be helpful as PD patients tend to have a slightly lower frequency tremor that can be difficult to distinguish in clinical practice. Dopamine-transporter single-photon emission computed tomography (DAT-SPECT) is a nuclear medicine study that uses a tracer for the dopamine transporter. This tracer can be used as a marker for dopaminergic nigrostriatal neurons. Patients with PD have decreased uptake compared to healthy controls and essential tremor patients, further favoring the diagnosis of tremor-dominant PD. However, this study is not foolproof as recent studies have suggested some degree of decreased uptake in patients with essential tremor as well. In the present case, DAT imaging showed significantly decreased uptake in favor of a diagnosis of PD (Figure 4.1).

Initial treatment for PD is always medical. Standard first-line therapy is with a dopamine agonist or monoamine oxidase (MAO) inhibitor in early stages and levodopa/carbidopa for later stages of the disease. Dopamine agonists are less effective than levodopa/carbidopa but are associated with fewer motor fluctuations. For this reason, they are used to delay the need to initiate levodopa therapy. Surgical consideration is typically reserved for patients who have begun to plateau on medical therapy or have developed side effects, most notably dyskinesias. This patient, like most patients referred

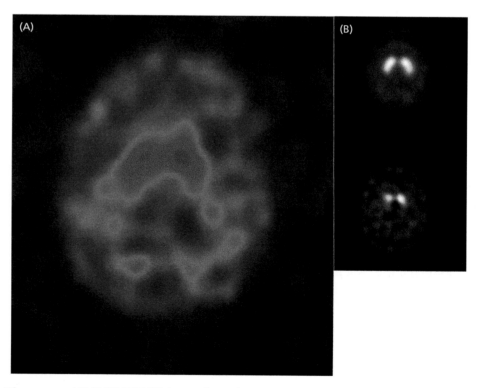

Figure 4.1 (A) DAT-SPECT image from this patient. (B) DAT-SPECT image of a patient without Parkinson disease (top) and one with severe Parkinson disease (bottom).

for potential surgical intervention, has already been established on a levodopa/carbidopa regimen and is currently developing motor fluctuation side effects.

Oral Boards Review—Diagnostic Pearls

Tremor-Dominant Parkinson Disease Versus Essential Tremor

	Parkinson Disease	Essential Tremor
Age of onset	Usually around 60 years old	Larger age variation (10–80 years old)
Family history	No	Yes
Tremor frequency	4–6 Hz	5–8 Hz
Rest tremor	Yes	In severe cases
Postural tremor	Presents after a delay	Presents without delay
Kinetic tremor	In severe cases	Yes
Tremor characteristics		
Symmetric	No	Yes
Resting	Worse	Better
Action	Better	Worse
Concentration	Better	Worse
Walking	Worse	Better
Writing	Better	Worse
Alcohol	No effect	Better
Other areas	Face, jaw	Head, voice
DAT-SPECT results	Marked deficit	Minimal deficit
Response to levodopa	Yes	No
Medical treatment	Dopamine, dopamine agonists, beta-blockers, primidone, alcohol, anticholinergics, MAO inhibitors, topiramate, gabapentin, Botox, amantadine	

Questions about anatomic/therapeutic details

1. Given the proposed diagnosis, what are the surgical treatment options?
2. What are potential surgical targets for this condition?
3. What factors would favor one surgical target over another?

Decision-Making

Surgical treatment options for advanced PD include implantation of a pump for continuous infusion of levodopa/carbidopa, typically enterally through the duodenum in a therapy known as Duodopa, and neurosurgical options. Duodopa has been shown to be effective in reducing the motor fluctuation associated with the otherwise-erratic absorption of oral levodopa therapy and is often the best choice for patients who are poor candidates for the more invasive neurosurgical options.

The neurosurgical options for treatment can be subdivided into either ablative or stimulation procedures. Ablative procedures are accomplished through either targeted radio frequency, gamma knife radiation, or more recently focused ultrasound. Stimulation procedures refer to deep brain stimulation (DBS), wherein a stimulating electrode is placed into either the basal ganglia or the thalamus. Several important differences exist between surgical treatments. Both DBS and radio-frequency ablation involve a scalp incision and small craniotomy for either the stimulating electrode or the radio-frequency probe. Microelectrode recording (MER) and subsequent stimulation in awake patients are classically used to precisely localize the target. Ablative procedures with either gamma knife or focused ultrasound cannot be done with MERs as neither procedure violates the scalp. Focused ultrasound procedures, however, do critically require the patient's hair to be shaved to allow adequate device penetration to the skin surface, whereas gamma knife procedures do not. Also, both ablative procedures are typically performed on an awake patient. This is particularly important for focused ultrasound, during which having an awake patient allows for detection of immediate benefit or side effects. With the gamma knife, however, this aspect of having an awake patient is not as significant because both benefit and side effects can take months to develop.

For tremor-dominant PD, the primary targeting question is between the ventral intermediate nucleus (VIM) of the thalamus versus the subthalamic nucleus (STN). The VIM thalamus is the target used for essential tremor, but it has also been shown to be highly effective in the treatment of Parkinsonian tremor, with favorable outcomes approaching 90%. Stimulation of the VIM thalamus has no effect on the other symptoms of PD, such as rigidity, bradykinesia, and gait abnormalities. The STN has been shown to reduce all of the motor effects of PD, though the initial reduction in tremor is not typically as impressive as it is with the VIM. In addition, there are neuropsychiatric sequelae from using the subthalamic nuclei. It is therefore avoided in patients who display a high risk of worsening neuropsychiatric outcome based on preoperative testing. On the other hand, for patients with bilateral symptoms, there is an increased risk of dysarthria or disequilibrium with bilateral VIM stimulation. For this reason, a unilateral-only procedure is utilized with this target.

Younger age tends to favor targeting of the STN as there is a high likelihood of developing both the other motor symptoms and motor fluctuations of the disease at a later stage. The thalamus is typically favored in older patients because the likelihood of developing additional symptoms or motor fluctuations is lower and the risk of neuropsychiatric complications of STN stimulation is higher.

Given this patient's age and additional motor symptoms, bilateral STN DBS was deemed the best next course of action by a multidisciplinary panel of neurologists, neurosurgeons, and neuropsychiatrists.

Questions

1. What are common techniques used for identifying the STN?
2. What are options in patients who cannot tolerate an awake procedure?

Surgical Procedure

Deep brain stimulation of the STN for PD is arguably the most common surgical procedure for a movement disorder. A variety of surgical techniques have been developed. The first step in all of these procedures involves identifying the approximate location of the dorsolateral portion of the STN on imaging, as this location in the STN has been shown to be most effective in symptomatic improvement. For tremor in particular, the most posterior portion of this region of STN is typically targeted. Magnetic resonance imaging (MRI) sequences, particularly three-dimensional, thin-cut, T1-weighted, and T2-weighted sequences through the basal ganglia and midbrain, are useful for this. Several variations of these sequences have been reported in the literature to better delineate the borders of the STN by different groups, but all typically involve both a T1 and T2 sequence. The T1 sequence is useful for identifying the anterior and posterior commissures. Once identified, indirect targeting of the STN can be done based on distance from the midcommissural point (MCP). For the STN, these coordinates are approximately 12 mm lateral, 4 mm posterior, and 4 mm inferior to the MCP. Further refinement can be done utilizing the red nucleus, which is usually visible on the T2-weighted sequence. The ideal location for STN stimulation is approximately 3 mm lateral and 2 mm below the anterolateral border of the red nucleus. In sequences where the borders of the STN are discernible, radiographic targeting can be even further refined using a variety of methods. These options include using a frame, having the patient awake, and performing MER. All variations in technique have been shown to be effective in the literature. The decision of which protocol to use ultimately rests on the comfort of the surgeon and the tolerance of the patient. For patients who cannot tolerate an awake procedure due to cognitive or psychological issues, intraoperative imaging is useful to confirm accurate positioning of the electrode prior to closure. This can be done either with intraoperative MRI, intraoperative computed tomography (CT) with subsequent fusion to preoperative planning images, or, in frame-based cases, with anteroposterior and lateral x-rays.

In awake cases, MER can be used to functionally delineate the top and bottom borders of the STN to allow for the most accurate placement of the electrode. This requires a degree of electrophysiological expertise from the surgeon, neurologist, or neurophysiologist. MERs can also be used in asleep cases, though activity of the STN can be significantly suppressed by anesthesia. Stimulation in awake cases also allows for further functional localization. For STN stimulation, paresthesia generated by stimulation at low-stimulation amplitudes suggests posteromedial placement affecting the medial meniscal fibers. Eye deviation further suggests a medially positioned electrode affecting the ipsilateral third nerve. Dysarthria and contractures of either the contralateral face or limbs suggests a placement that is too anterolateral with internal capsule involvement. Of note, transient paresthesia of the contralateral limb or face with high amplitudes can suggest good placement of the electrode.

This patient underwent bilateral STN DBS using a frame, MER, and intraoperative stimulation.

Oral Boards Review—Management Pearls

1. The indirect target for the STN is 12 mm lateral, 4 mm posterior, and 4 mm inferior to the MCP.
2. With stimulation, both the response in symptoms and the generated side effects are useful to functionally locate the electrode position.
3. Significant improvement in symptoms at low amplitudes with transient paresthesia of the contralateral limb at high amplitudes (higher than what would be used in therapy) that resolves over time indicates ideal electrode placement.

Pivot Points

1. If the patient has any sign of a poor neurocognitive status, full neuropsychiatric testing should be performed. If there is a verified deficit, the STN should be avoided as a stimulation target due to risk of cognitive decline after surgery.
2. If neurocognitive status is a concern, either the VIM thalamus or the globus pallidus internus (GPi) could be used. Data on stimulation of the GPi suggest that it is practically as effective in reducing Parkinsonian tremor as the STN, though it might be slightly less effective in reducing levodopa dosages, bradykinesia, and rigidity. It is, however, better at improving medication-associated dyskinesias.

Aftercare

After intracranial electrode placement, patients are usually monitored overnight for potentially devastating perioperative complications, such as hemorrhage or stroke. This is typically performed in an intensive care unit or at least intermediate care unit. A postoperative scan is performed to confirm adequate placement of the electrode, and the patient is usually mobilized the same day. If a Foley catheter was placed during the procedure, it is removed the day of mobilization. Prophylactic postoperative antibiotics are not typically given as there is no strong evidence to suggest that they reduce the rate of infection.

Placement of the battery can be done on the same day as the electrode placement or at a later date. In either case, the tunneling portion of the procedure to connect the extension cables to the battery is painful and requires general anesthesia. If the procedure is staged on different days, this second stage is typically done in an outpatient surgery setting.

Postoperatively, there is a period of benefit from the microlesioning effect that can last from a few days to several months. The battery is not activated during this period to preserve as much energy as possible. Once symptoms return, the initial programming session is typically done by the neurologist. Patients should be counseled that it may take up to 6 months to achieve optimal programming and benefit of the device.

Complications and Management

Infection is the most common complication following DBS for tremor-dominant PD and occurs in approximately 5% of cases. Battery replacements also have around a 5% risk of infection. The generator pocket is the most common site in most studies. Generator site infection is usually managed by removal of the generator, wound washout, and intravenous antibiotics for upward of 6 weeks. When a lead or cranial incision is involved, the entire system must also be removed. However, in superficial infections of the generator site, antibiotics alone can also be a feasible strategy.

Other complications, including lead migration, hemorrhage, or stroke, are less frequent. Mortality risk is low during this procedure. Management for lead migration usually requires revision surgery for replacement. For hemorrhage and stroke, most cases are asymptomatic and incidentally found on postoperative imaging. However, in cases with associated neurological decline, surgery can be necessary. Ablative procedures are associated with higher rates of neurological deficits, which can be permanent. However, they are also generally associated with lower infection rates because no permanent hardware is implanted.

Oral Boards Review—Complications Pearls

1. Infection is the most common complication from DBS, though neurological deficits are also a possibility. Ablative procedures involve a lower risk of infection but a higher risk of neurological deficits.
2. Infection in DBS cases should be treated with removal of the affected portion of the system and intravenous antibiotics. In rare situations of superficial pocket infections, an antibiotic alone is a feasible option.

Evidence and Outcomes

There is strong evidence supporting DBS of either the VIM or STN in the treatment of Parkinsonian tremor. There is much less evidence comparing the efficacy of targets, but early retrospective analysis showed no significant difference in tremor reduction between the two sites. As mentioned previously, STN stimulation is better than VIM stimulation for improving other motor symptoms aside from tremor. Ablative strategies have also been shown to have efficacy in reducing tremor but are associated with increased neurological side effects.

References and Further Reading

1. Stebbins, G. T., et al. How to identify tremor dominant and postural instability/gait difficulty groups with the movement disorder society unified Parkinson's disease rating scale: comparison with the unified Parkinson's disease rating scale: PIGD and The MDS-UPDRS. *Mov Disord.* **28**, 668–670 (2013). http://www.ncbi.nlm.nih.gov/pubmed/23408503
2. Thenganatt, M. A., & Louis, E. D. Distinguishing essential tremor from Parkinson's disease: bedside tests and laboratory evaluations. *Expert Rev Neurother.* **12**, 687–696 (2012). http://www.ncbi.nlm.nih.gov/pubmed/22650171

3. Jankovic, J. Parkinson's disease: clinical features and diagnosis. *J Neurol Neurosurg Psychiatry* **79**, 368–376 (2008). http://www.ncbi.nlm.nih.gov/pubmed/18344392

4. Connolly, B. S., & Lang, A. E. Pharmacological treatment of Parkinson disease: a review. *JAMA* **311**, 1670 (2014). http://www.ncbi.nlm.nih.gov/pubmed/24756517

5. Volkmann, J., Daniels, C., & Witt, K. Neuropsychiatric effects of subthalamic neurostimulation in Parkinson disease. *Nat Rev Neurol* **6**, 487–498 (2010). http://www.ncbi.nlm.nih.gov/pubmed/20680036

6. Parihar, R., Alterman, R., Papavassiliou, E., Tarsy, D., and Shih, L. Comparison of VIM and STN DBS for Parkinsonian resting and postural/action tremor. *Tremor Other Hyperkinet Mov (NY)* **5**, 321 (2015). doi:10.7916/d81v5d35. http://www.ncbi.nlm.nih.gov/pubmed/26196027

7. Fraix, V., Pollak, P., Moro, E., Chabardes, S., Xie, J., Ardouin, C., and Benabid, A.L. Subthalamic nucleus stimulation in tremor dominant Parkinsonian patients with previous thalamic surgery. *J Neurol Neurosurg Psychiatry* **76**, 246–248 (2005). http://www.ncbi.nlm.nih.gov/pubmed/15654041

8. Perestelo-Pérez, L., et al. Deep brain stimulation in Parkinson's disease: meta-analysis of randomized controlled trials. *J Neurol* **261**, 2051–2060 (2014). https://www.ncbi.nlm.nih.gov/pubmed/24487826

Obsessive-Compulsive Disorder

Patrick J. Karas and Ashwin Viswanathan

5

Case Presentation

A 36-year-old woman with severe treatment-refractory obsessive-compulsive disorder (OCD) presents to your clinic for surgical consultation. She was diagnosed with OCD 11 years ago at age 25, shortly after losing her job as a paralegal. She has severe anxiety involving maintaining cleanliness around her workspace. While keeping tidy had always been a point of pride for her, she gradually became fixated on the idea that the papers on her desk were not ordered correctly and were contaminated. While she knows she has repeatedly checked and found everything to be satisfactory, she continues to sort through her papers for hours a day in an attempt to relieve her anxiety. She has been treated with several selective serotonin reuptake inhibitors (SSRIs), venlafaxine, buspirone, and lithium and has undergone repeated trials of cognitive behavioral therapy (CBT) with good compliance. Despite years of treatment, she continues to have significant impairment. She also states she frequently has depressed mood in addition to difficulty sleeping and anhedonia. Her accompanying records state her current Yale-Brown Obsessive Compulsive Scale (YBOCS) is 31. Other than her psychiatric illness, she has no medical or surgical history. She was referred to you by her managing psychiatrist for consideration of deep brain stimulation (DBS).

Questions

1. What are the different surgical treatments for OCD?
2. How is OCD severity scored?
3. What are the targets for surgical intervention in OCD?
4. What is the current theory for the pathophysiology of OCD?
5. What are contraindications to surgical intervention?
6. What is the efficacy of DBS for OCD?

Assessment and Planning

Obsessive-compulsive disorder is a phenotypically heterogeneous psychiatric disorder affecting 1%–2% of the US population. Typically treated with medication and behavioral therapy, roughly 20%–30% of people suffering from OCD have severe, refractory symptoms despite maximal medical and behavioral treatments. Thus, there remains significant unmet need from people suffering from severe refractory OCD (>600,000 people in the United States).

Deep brain stimulation of the bilateral anterior limb of the internal capsule (ALIC) received a Food and Drug Administration (FDA) Humanitarian Device Exemption (HDE) in 2009 for patients with severe treatment-refractory OCD. Prior to approval for DBS, the only surgical treatments for severe OCD that were medication and behavioral therapy resistant were ablative procedures such as anterior cingulotomy and anterior capsulotomy.

Diagnosis of OCD is performed according to *Diagnostic and Statistical Manual of Mental Disorders* (*DSM*; currently the fifth edition [*DSM-5*]). OCD is a psychiatric disorder defined by intrusive and distressing thoughts (obsessions), often coupled with repetitive physical or mental routines (compulsions). Obsessions are usually the cause of anxiety to sufferers, and the compulsions manifest as attempts by the patient to control distress. Patients typically have good insight, realizing the obsessions or compulsions are excessive. Moreover, many patients even understand the compulsions do not meaningfully address the obsessions. Importantly, the *DSM-5* diagnostic criteria necessitate that the obsessions/compulsions significantly interfere with the patient's life, manifesting through diverse means, such as academic, professional, or interpersonal avenues.

The OCD manifestations can be very phenotypically heterogeneous. Two patients diagnosed with OCD may have completely different manifestations of their obsessions or compulsions. As anatomically distinct brain regions may govern this phenotypic diversity, patient selection for surgical treatment remains an area of study. Moreover, there may not be a "best" target that effectively treats all patients with OCD. To this end, phenotypic diversity of the disorder has been characterized. Obsessions can be divided into subtypes centered on symmetry, taboo (aggressive or sexual) thoughts, contamination (dirt), and hoarding. While subtypes or obsessions are frequently associated with typical compulsions, some patients do not experience compulsions. Adding to this phenotypic diversity is time of onset. In 30%–50% of cases, onset occurs during childhood. In fact, several studies question if pediatric and adult-onset OCD have the same underlying pathophysiology.

Obsessive-compulsive disorder is diagnosed and treated by psychiatrists, and the specifics of diagnosis and management are outside the scope of standard neurosurgical practice. Severity of OCD is rated according to the YBOCS. The scale scores symptom severity over five dimensions: (1) time occupied; (2) degree of difficulty functioning or with relationships; (3) distress; (4) resistance to obsessions/compulsions; and (5) success with resistance and control over symptoms. While a maximum score is 40, scores above 24 are characterized as "severe," and scores above 32 are "extreme." In published trials, 28 is often the minimum cutoff to be considered for surgical intervention.

Standard treatment for OCD is multimodal therapy, including serotonergic antidepressants and CBT. Prior to consideration for surgery, a patient must fail conventional treatment. Failure, defined by inclusion criteria in clinical trials to date, includes trial without symptomatic relief of at least three different serotonin reuptake inhibitors at 10 weeks of the maximum tolerated dose, failure of supplementation of serotonin reuptake inhibitors with neuroleptics and benzodiazepines (e.g., buspirone, lithium, or clonazepam), as well as failure through completion of at least 20 hours of behavioral therapy. While practices vary, a conservative approach also requires uncontrolled OCD to be present for 5 years prior to consideration for surgical intervention.

Assessment for implantation of DBS electrodes is a multidisciplinary endeavor, requiring partnership between neurosurgeon and treating psychiatrist. In addition to patient selection, a psychiatrist must agree to follow a patient for continuation of medical and behavioral treatment after surgery, in addition to management of DBS stimulation settings.

Common comorbidities of OCD include anxiety, depression, tic disorders (particularly in children), attention deficit hyperactivity disorder (ADHD), and other neurodevelopmental disorders. It is imperative that these comorbid psychiatric disorders be discussed with the patient's referring/treating psychiatrist prior to proceeding with surgery. Caution should be used when considering surgical intervention in patients with substance abuse disorders, psychotic or manic episodes, or severe personality disorders, as these disorders are associated with decreased efficacy or worsening of psychiatric side effects.

As for any elective cranial surgery, standard presurgical medical assessment is required. Patients undergoing DBS for OCD tend to be younger than their cohorts undergoing DBS for Parkinson disease or essential tremor. However, medical clearance, optimization of comorbid medical problems, and detailed review of medical and psychiatric history are essential prior to surgery. Antiplatelet and anticoagulation medications need to be held or fully reversed prior to surgery. Surgical staging is at the discretion of the surgeon and patient; like in DBS for indications other than OCD, surgery can be completed in one or two stages.

Oral Boards Review—Diagnostic Pearls

1. OCD is a psychiatric illness characterized by recurrent intrusive thoughts and impulses, often coupled with ritualized, repetitive, compulsive behaviors aimed at allaying the patient's anxiety. Despite often understanding that their obsessions and compulsions are irrational and excessive, patients are significantly impaired in daily life.
2. Because the diagnosis and treatment of OCD is out of the scope of standard neurosurgical practice, it is imperative that surgical assessment of patients with OCD be performed in close partnership with the patient's treating psychiatrist. Furthermore, a psychiatrist must continue to care for the patient after surgery.
3. Standard treatment of OCD includes SSRIs in addition to CBT. Prior to consideration for surgery, a patient must fail behavioral therapy as well as multiple trials of SSRIs, supplemented with antidopaminergic, neuroleptic, or benzodiazepine treatment.
4. Severity of OCD is rated according to the YBOCS. A minimum score of 28 despite maximum medical and behavioral therapy is required prior to consideration for surgical treatment. The maximum score is 40.

Questions

1. What are the clinical symptoms of OCD?
2. What are the standard pharmacologic and behavioral treatments for OCD?
3. What clinical criteria must a patient meet prior to consideration for surgery for OCD?

Decision-Making

Precise targeting for DBS lead placement remains a subject of debate due to lack of understanding of the exact mechanisms underlying OCD, phenotypic heterogeneity (and therefore possible neural mechanistic heterogeneity), and lack of differentiation in clinical efficacy between different stimulation targets. It must be emphasized that presently FDA HDE approval is specific to bilateral ALIC stimulation; thus, other stimulation targets remain investigational. In addition to ALIC, other stimulation targets include the ventral striatum/ventral capsule (VS/VC), nucleus accumbens (NAc), subthalamic nucleus (STN), bed nucleus of striae terminalis (BST), and inferior thalamic peduncle (ITP). As many of these structures are adjacent (or within millimeters), more than one of these targets may be stimulated with thoughtful lead trajectory and depth of lead placement. Exact coordinates for stimulation targets continue to be revised as new trials are published.

Stimulation targets were initially chosen based on experience from a long history of ablative procedures for OCD. The majority of DBS targets (ALIC, VC/VS, and ITP) derive from anterior capsulotomy, a procedure that destroys white matter tracts traveling between the prefrontal cortex and subcortical nuclei (most notably the dorsomedial thalamus). Other ablative procedures for OCD include anterior cingulotomy, currently without DBS correlate, which creates a lesion at the juncture of cingulate cortical gray matter and the cingulum white matter tract. Another ablative procedure, subcaudate tractotomy, lesions the substantia innominata, an area just below the anterior thalamus and head of caudate that contains white matter tracts connecting the orbitofrontal cortex (OFC) to subcortical nuclei. Importantly, the gamma knife is increasingly being used to perform these ablative procedures in place of thermal lesioning.

In addition to understanding the surgical predecessors to DBS for OCD, an understanding of the current theories for the pathophysiology of OCD is helpful in identifying proper stimulation targets. OCD arises from imbalances in a complex combination of serotonergic, dopaminergic, and glutamatergic transmissions through cortico-striato-thalamo-cortical (CSTC) feedback loops. Abnormal neurotransmitter activity ultimately leads to hyperactivity of the anterior cingulate cortex (ACC) and medial and lateral OFC. The medial OFC is involved in behavioral reinforcement as well as stimulus-reward association, while the lateral OFC mediates behavior reversal and conflict resolution. The ACC is thought to perform error monitoring and activates in situations of complex decision-making.

Pathologically elevated OFC and ACC activity is mediated through an imbalance between direct and indirect CSTC pathways, specifically overactivation of the direct pathway out of proportion to the indirect pathway (Figure 5.1). In the direct pathway, striatal activation from the OFC and ACC increases gamma-aminobutyric acid–ergic

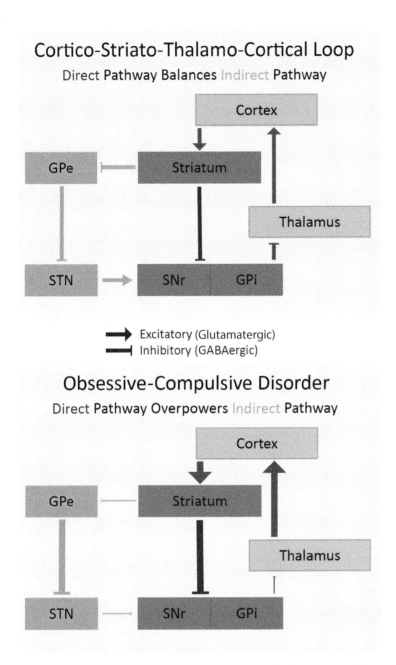

Figure 5.1 In the normally functioning cortico-striato-thalamo-cortical circuit, direct (purple) and indirect (orange) pathways lead to increased or decreased inhibition of the thalamus, respectively, in a balanced manner. In obsessive-compulsive disorder (OCD), overactivation of the direct pathway out of proportion to the indirect pathway leads to pathologic overactivity of cortical regions in an insidious excitatory loop. GPe, globus pallidus externa; GPi, globus pallidus interna; SNr, substantia nigra pars reticulata; STN, subthalamic nucleus.

(GABAergic) inhibitory stimulation of the globus pallidus interna (GPi) and substantia nigra pars reticulata (SNr). Elevated inhibition of the GPi and SNr decreases inhibitory GABAergic stimuli from these nuclei onto the thalamus, causing increased excitatory glutamatergic stimulation from the thalamus back onto the OFC and ACC. Thus the direct pathway is a positive feedforward loop where activation of the OFC and ACC leads to more activation of these same cortical regions.

In contrast, the indirect pathway is an inhibitory feedback loop. Excitatory glutamatergic signals from the OFC and ACC onto the striatum increase inhibitory GABAergic signals from the striatum to the globus pallidus externa (GPe). Decreased GPe activity in turn decreases inhibition of the STN, causing a net increase in GPi and SNr activity. Since the GPi and SNr pass inhibitory GABAergic signals to the thalamus, thalamic activity is decreased by the indirect pathway, ultimately decreasing activity of the OFC and ACC. Overactivation of the direct pathway, out of proportion to the indirect pathway, is thought to lead to the increased OFC and ACC activity characteristic of OCD.

Deep brain stimulation and lesioning procedures are thought to interrupt the abnormal positive feedback of the direct CSTC loop described previously. Hyperactivity of the OFC has been observed to decrease in a manner correlating strongly with treatment effect after surgery, a finding similar to that which occurs after successful treatment with serotonergic medications. However, the exact way in which surgery modifies the balance between direct and indirect pathways is unclear.

Questions

1. For which anatomic target(s) does DBS for OCD have FDA HDE?
2. What cortical regions are thought to play a role in the pathophysiology of OCD?
3. Describe the direct and indirect pathways of the CSTC loop thought to play a role in the pathophysiology of OCD.

Surgical Procedure

Selection of the anatomical target for electrode placement is performed before surgery. Stereotactic planning for lead placement should also be done prior to surgery. Preoperative T2 magnetic resonance imaging (MRI) is used for target identification and lead placement. MRI sequences such as fast gray matter acquisition T1 inversion recovery (FGATIR) are being developed to increase subcortical structure contrast to improve lead placement. It is also important to ask patients their preference for battery placement site and laterality prior to surgery.

As previously mentioned, optimal intracranial electrode placement remains an area of active study. Here we discuss recommended lead placement for ALIC/BST and VC/VS stimulation. The ALIC and BST target is 1–2 mm posterior to the anterior commissure (AC), at the junction of the AC and ALIC (Figure 5.2). Electrode zero is placed 1–2 mm deep to the axial anterior commissure/posterior commissure (AC/PC) plane and 7 mm from the midline. It is important to plan a trajectory where the electrodes

Axial	Coronal	Sagittal

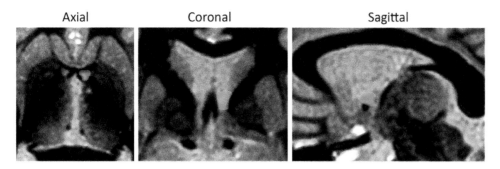

Figure 5.2 Fast gray matter acquisition T1 inversion recovery (FGATIR) sequence in three planes: axial, sagittal, and coronal (1 mm posterior to the posterior aspect of the anterior commissure). The bed nucleus of the stria terminalis is highlighted in blue and is bounded laterally by the internal capsule and medially by the fornix.

follow the course of the ALIC in the coronal plane so that the lead lays in the BST just dorsal to the AC.

Alternatively, the VC/VS target is in the VS, with electrode zero just deep to the axial AC/PC plane. In a study rating efficacy based on lead placement, optimum targeting was 6–8 mm from the midline, 0–2 mm anterior to the AC, and 3–4 mm ventral to the AC/PC plane. Again it is important to plan a trajectory following the course of the internal capsule so that electrodes one and two lay in the ventral half of the internal capsule, and contact 3 lays at the dorsal margin of the internal capsule.

Leads are placed under stereotactic guidance. Choice of frame-based systems such as Leksell (Elekta, Stockholm, Sweden) and CRW (Integra LifeSciences, Plainsboro, NJ) or frameless systems such as NexFrame (Medtronic, Minneapolis, MN) and STarFix (FHC, Bowdoin, ME) is based on availability and surgeon preference. We prefer stereotactic frame placement and use an intraoperative O-arm (Medtronic) obtained after frame placement for registration with the preoperative MRI.

Notably, because stimulator leads must run along the course of the ALIC to the anatomic target, burr-hole placement must be planned with stereotaxy after intracranial lead placement planning is complete. Burr-hole sites should be marked, then the patient can be prepped and draped for surgery. After burr holes are made, hemostasis is essential prior to dural opening. Losing a large volume of cerebrospinal fluid (CSF) can lead to brain sag and shift, causing errors in stereotaxy. Therefore, minimizing dural openings helps to avoid excessive CSF loss. CSF loss can also be minimized by filling burr holes with a fibrin sealant after cannula placement. To minimize cortical damage and the risk of bleeding, cortical veins should be avoided. The brain cannula should be placed perpendicular to a gyrus surface, and sulci should also be avoided. The cortical surface should be bipolared and sharply incised with a blade prior to introducing a cannula. The blood pressure should also be well controlled to prevent tract hemorrhage, maintaining systolic blood pressure below 140 mm Hg. Electrodes should not take a transventricular route as transventricular placement is associated with greater CSF loss and intraventricular hemorrhage. Finally, cortical and tract hemorrhage can be minimized by avoiding multiple cannula/microelectrode/stimulation lead passes.

As is common practice during electrode placement in DBS for other indications, the patient should be awakened during surgery for intraoperative stimulation. Intraoperative testing is particularly important for OCD given the variety of anatomic targets and landmarks for electrode placement, allowing for testing both efficacy and side-effect tolerance. A sensation of mirth on stimulation has been correlated with good treatment response and can be used as an intraoperative indicator of proper placement. On the contrary, eliciting a response of fear or anxiety, particularly on activation of the deepest electrode, may indicate that the electrode is too deep. Intraoperative microelectrode recording remains investigational and does not currently aid placement.

Once the stimulation leads are placed in the correct position, the leads are locked in place with a specially designed burr-hole cover. The remaining wires are tunneled under the skin to the side where the battery is to be placed. Battery placement, considered stage 2 of the procedure, can occur on the same day or after recovery from the cranial procedure.

Oral Boards Review—Management Pearls

1. Avoiding intraoperative hypertension and minimizing intraoperative CSF drainage are essential technical aspects to minimize the occurrence of intracranial hemorrhage and avoid missing the intracranial lead targets.
2. Close partnership with a patient's psychiatrist is necessary when undertaking DBS for OCD. It is often helpful for the psychiatrist to be present in the operating room for assistance with intraoperative stimulation testing.

Pivot Points

1. If a new neurologic deficit manifests during surgery, the surgery should be promptly aborted and the patient taken for stat computed tomography of the head.
2. While intraoperative stimulation testing can help to avoid undesirable stimulation side effects (anxiety, fear), failing to elicit desired responses (mirth, joy) in the operating room should not be an indication to abort the procedure.

Aftercare

Patients are generally observed overnight after placement of intracranial electrodes and are discharged on postoperative day 1 in uncomplicated cases. The patient should be scheduled to see his or her psychiatrist approximately 2 weeks after completion of surgery, at which time the electrodes can be turned on and initial programming can take place.

Complications and Management

Complications can be divided into two broad categories: surgical complications and stimulation side effects. Surgical complications are those inherent to DBS surgery, including infection, hemorrhage, and seizure. Risk of hemorrhage is 1%–3%, with increased risk with advanced patient age, transventricular or trans-sulcal electrode trajectory, and hypertension (particularly intraoperative). Wound complications, including infection, CSF leak, or device erosion, occur in roughly 5% of cases. Infections involving hardware necessitate removal of the involved section of hardware followed by antibiotic treatment. Removal of intracranial electrodes carries a risk of intracranial hemorrhage. Occurrence of seizure (1%–2%) and subdural hematoma (1%–2%) are other surgical complications. Routine perioperative seizure prophylaxis is not common practice. Risk of subdural hematoma can be minimized by meticulous sharp incision of pia prior to electrode insertion to prevent sheering of cortical veins. Perioperative mortality rates are similar compared to other elective cranial procedures, and rates can be minimized with proper preoperative evaluation and medical optimization. Patients should be mobilized as soon as possible after surgery (on the day of surgery or postoperative day 1), and postoperative care should include standard practices, such as incentive spirometry, early discontinuation of a Foley catheter, and so on.

Stimulation side effects can occur immediately or in delayed fashion after the stimulator is activated. Effects can vary greatly, including sensory changes (taste and smell); autonomic symptoms (diaphoresis, tachypnea, hot or cold sensations); and mood changes (fear, panic, sadness, or elation). For some patients, improvement in mood can be a positive side effect; however, for other patients mood change can present as hypomania. Fortunately these undesired effects stop after termination of stimulation. Importantly, just as undesired effects cease with termination of stimulation, patients can experience acute severe recurrent OCD on interruption of stimulation from malfunction or battery depletion. A nonnegligible number of patients with OCD have reported uncomfortable feelings of the hardware under their skin, requiring subsequent hardware removal. Delayed occurrence of seizures has also been reported after chronic stimulation, though the incidence of this is unclear.

Oral Boards Review—Complications Pearls

1. Meticulous attention to hemostasis, preventing excess CSF runoff, and blood pressure at the time of cortical electrode placement helps to prevent hemorrhage and poor electrode placement.
2. It is imperative that hardware be regularly monitored, as battery failure can lead to acute exacerbation of OCD symptoms.

Evidence and Outcomes

While stimulation of the ALIC has the largest body of evidence, none of the previously discussed anatomic targets has been proven superior. Because ALIC and VC/VS have the most evidence, we focus on those outcomes. Treatment response is defined as greater than 35% reduction in YBOCS compared to preoperative baseline, a benchmark borrowed from pharmaceutical trials in OCD.

The largest series of ALIC stimulation to date followed 24 patients with severe treatment-resistant OCD in an open-label trial, with 17 of those patients undergoing crossover (on vs. off or off vs. on) stimulation. Of the patients, 53% achieved treatment response at crossover (median 63% reduction in YBOCS among responders,

$n = 17$). Also, 67% responded at last follow-up (median improvement 58% in YBOCS reduction; last follow-up 15–171 months, median 72 months, $n = 24$). The authors then analyzed outcome based on electrode positioning, determining that response rates improved to 67% at crossover and 83% at last follow-up if stimulation included the BST.

The largest single series of VC/VS stimulation followed 10 patients. Of these patients, 50% ($n = 4$) achieved treatment response at 36 months, with an additional 25% of patients obtaining 25%–35% reduction in YBOCS. In a combined study from four sites, follow-up data from 26 patients implanted with VC/VS were reviewed. Of patients, 48% responded to treatment at 12 months ($n = 21$), 58% of patients were responders at 36 months ($n = 12$), and 62% at last follow-up ($n = 26$, last follow-up 3–36 months, mean 31.4 months). The authors also analyzed lead placement, finding treatment response improved to 75% at last follow-up in patients with more posterior electrode targeting.

In summary, across ALIC/BST and VC/VS studies, roughly 50% of patients responded to treatment, achieving at least 35% reduction in YBOCS after stimulation. These results are similar to results for traditional ablative procedures, with the advantage that stimulation effects are reversible. Because many aspects of DBS for OCD, including proper patient selection and optimal electrode placement, are still under active investigation. Neurosurgeons undertaking this procedure are recommended to contribute to surgical literature with careful review of patient outcomes.

References and Further Reading

De Koning, P. P., Figee, M., Van Den Munckhof, P., Schuurman, P. R., & Denys, D. (2011). Current status of deep brain stimulation for obsessive-compulsive disorder: a clinical review of different targets. *Current Psychiatry Reports*, *13*(4), 274–282. https://doi.org/10.1007/s11920-011-0200-8

Greenberg, B. D., Gabriels, L. A., Malone, D. A., Rezai, A. R., Friehs, G. M., Okun, M. S., . . . Nuttin, B. J. (2010). Deep brain stimulation of the ventral internal capsule/ventral striatum for obsessive-compulsive disorder: worldwide experience. *Molecular Psychiatry*, *15*(1), 64–79. https://doi.org/10.1038/mp.2008.55

Greenberg, B. D., Rauch, S. L., & Haber, S. N. (2010). Invasive circuitry-based neurotherapeutics: stereotactic ablation and deep brain stimulation for OCD. *Neuropsychopharmacology: Official Publication of the American College of Neuropsychopharmacology*, *35*(1), 317–336. https://doi.org/10.1038/npp.2009.128

Luyten, L., Hendrickx, S., Raymaekers, S., Gabriëls, L., & Nuttin, B. (2016). Electrical stimulation in the bed nucleus of the stria terminalis alleviates severe obsessive-compulsive disorder. *Molecular Psychiatry*, *21*(9), 1272–1280. https://doi.org/10.1038/mp.2015.124

Okun, M. S., Mann, G., Foote, K. D., Shapira, N. A., Bowers, D., Springer, U., . . . Goodman, W. K. (2007). Deep brain stimulation in the internal capsule and nucleus accumbens region: responses observed during active and sham programming. *Journal of Neurology, Neurosurgery, and Psychiatry*, *78*(3), 310–314. https://doi.org/10.1136/jnnp.2006.095315

Pauls, D. L., Abramovitch, A., Rauch, S. L., & Geller, D. A. (2014). Obsessive-compulsive disorder: an integrative genetic and neurobiological perspective. *Nature Reviews Neuroscience*, *15*(6), 410–424. https://doi.org/10.1038/nrn3746

Raymaekers, S., Vansteelandt, K., Luyten, L., Bervoets, C., Demyttenaere, K., Gabriëls, L., & Nuttin, B. (2016). Long-term electrical stimulation of bed nucleus of stria terminalis for obsessive-compulsive disorder. *Molecular Psychiatry*, *22*(February), 1–4. https://doi.org/10.1038/mp.2016.124

Hypothalamic Hamartoma Causing Gelastic Seizures

Nisha Giridharan, Patrick J. Karas, and Daniel J. Curry

6

Case Presentation

A 9-year-old right-handed boy presents to your clinic for complaints of odd behavior. His mother states that he was diagnosed with seizures 2 years ago. He has several seizure types. During the most frequent types, he feels a good sensation then becomes glassy-eyed with uncharacteristic laughter lasting for a few seconds followed by a return to baseline. These happen sporadically, sometimes more than once a day and sometimes weeks apart. A second, less frequent, seizure begins similarly to the first type but is followed by swallowing and repetitive twisting and extension of the upper extremities lasting 5–30 seconds. These episodes are followed by sleepiness, and he usually sleeps for several hours. His mother states that in retrospect, even prior to diagnosis, he had always been a giggly baby. He was never treated with antiepileptic medications; his mother was told that medications would not help his type of seizures.

He was born full term with no complications, and his development to date has been normal. He is currently in second grade and performing normally in school. He does have occasional behavioral problems, with rare inconsolable fits of rage. There is no family history of epilepsy. On examination, his appearance, behavior, speech, and cognitive function appear normal for his age. He has no focal neurologic deficits. Neuropsychological testing is normal except for mild impairment in visuospatial function.

Magnetic resonance imaging (MRI) shows a nonenhancing, 9-mm T1 isointense mass protruding into the third ventricle from adjacent to the anterior pillars of the fornix (Figure 6.1). The boy's mother states that she wants treatment for his seizures; she was told that surgery is the best option.

Questions

1. What is the most likely diagnosis?
2. What other clinical features would raise suspicion for this diagnosis?
3. What imaging should be acquired?
4. What is an electroencephalogram (EEG) likely to show?
5. Would you recommend surgery? If so, what kind?

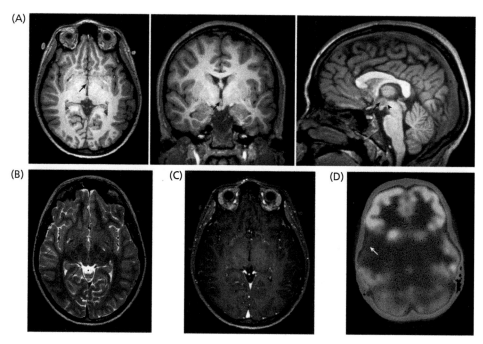

Figure 6.1 Preoperative imaging. (A) T1 noncontrast MRI in axial, coronal, and sagittal planes. There is a right-sided, 9-mm diameter, sessile, Delalande type 2 hypothalamic hamartoma (black arrow) extending into the inferior third ventricle. The hamartoma is isointense to gray matter on T1 imaging. Note how the right mammillothalamic tract wraps posteriorly around the hamartoma on the sagittal image (black arrowhead). (B) T2 axial MRI remonstrating the isointense to slightly hyperintense hamartoma. (C) T1 axial postcontrast MRI demonstrating no contrast enhancement of the hypothalamic hamartoma. (D) Fluorodeoxyglucose positron emission tomography (FDG-PET) demonstrates decreased FDG activity in the right middle and anterior temporal lobe (white arrow). This decreased activity may be reflective of secondary epileptogenesis; however, the hypothalamic hamartoma remains the primary epileptogenic lesion and must always be addressed first.

Assessment and Planning

Hypothalamic hamartomas (HHs) are rare, largely sporadic, lesions occurring in 1 in every 200,000 to 600,000 people. HH lesions are benign, heterotopic masses that occur due to anomalies in neuronal migration. Grossly they appear like normal brain parenchyma arising from the tuber cinereum and floor of the third ventricle. Microscopically, HHs consist of well-differentiated neuronal cells and glia.

The most common clinical manifestations of HH are central precocious puberty (CPP) and epilepsy, with gelastic (laughing) and dacrystic (crying) seizures comprising the most common seizure phenotype. Gelastic seizures are characterized by stereotyped, emotionless bursts of laughter or grimacing. Dacrystic seizures, less common than gelastic seizures, bear more resemblance to crying but can manifest as odd combinations of laughter and cries. While gelastic and dacrystic seizures are most often associated with HH, these seizure types can also rarely manifest in patients with frontal or temporal lobe epilepsies as well as focal cortical dysplasia, tuberous sclerosis, and tumor-related seizures.

The presence of either CPP or gelastic seizures, particularly when diagnosed early in childhood, should raise suspicion for HH, and diagnostic imaging with high-resolution MRI should be pursued.

Advances in MRI quality have improved the diagnosis of HHs. HH lesions are isointense on T1-weighted MR sequences, slightly hyperintense on T2 MRIs, and do not enhance after gadolinium administration. Magnetic resonance (MR) spectroscopy of HH tissue shows a significantly reduced N-acetylaspartate/creatinine ratio, with an increase in choline/creatinine ratio compared to normal hypothalamus. Increased myoinositol is also seen in HH, suggestive of higher levels of gliosis compared to surrounding gray matter.

The HHs have been traditionally classified into two morphologies based on imaging: sessile and pedunculated. Lesions are defined as sessile if the base of the mass partially or completely attaches to the third ventricle, often with distortion or displacement of surrounding structures, such as mammillary bodies. In contrast, pedunculated tumors are suspended from the floor of the third ventricle down into the suprasellar cistern by a small tissue attachment. Location of the HH in the anterior-posterior plane is often associated with the presenting symptom. HHs located anteriorly near the tuber cinereum are more associated with CPP, likely due to disturbance to the anteriorly located sexually dimorphic nuclei in the medial preoptic area of the hypothalamus that govern gonadotropin release. Lesions located posteriorly near the mammillary bodies and anterior pillars of the fornix are more typically associated with epilepsy. Abnormal electrical activity is thought to spread from hamartomatous tissue through the mammillary bodies/mammillothalamic tract through the Papez circuit to the mesial temporal lobe. Manifestations of laughter are triggered by propagation of the seizure down the dorsal longitudinal fasciculus to the nucleus retroambiguous in the medulla. Large HHs can be associated with both CPP and epilepsy.

The HHs are intrinsically epileptogenic. Epileptogenicity has been confirmed with depth electrode studies recording seizure onset from hamartomatous tissue. Moreover, stimulation of electrodes within HHs elicits habitual gelastic seizures. Additional evidence of intrinsic epileptogenicity comes from both fluorodeoxyglucose positron emission tomographic (FDG-PET) studies demonstrating glucose hypermetabolism in some HH lesions and functional MRI studies showing blood oxygen level–dependent activation of peri-HH tissue during clinical seizures. Scalp EEG patterns are often nonspecific for gelastic seizures. Recordings can capture slow spike and wave epileptiform discharges arising from frontal or temporal lobes, but seizure onset in deep structures such as the hypothalamus are not well recorded with scalp EEG.

Gelastic epilepsy related to HHs is typically refractory to medication. As such, secondary epileptogenesis in patients with HH is common, manifesting clinically as the development of secondary seizure types, epileptic encephalopathy, and clinical deterioration as children reach school age. Early neurosurgical intervention can help prevent secondary epileptogenesis as well as the progressive behavioral and cognitive decline associated with HHs.

Children and young adults can also have other nonepileptic manifestations of HH, such as behavior disturbance (rage attacks), hypothalamic obesity, and impaired cognition.

In the present case, MRI of the brain demonstrated a 9-mm, nonenhancing, isointense mass extending from the right floor of the third ventricle, adjacent to the mammillary body and into the interpeduncular cistern (Figure 6.1A–C). An EEG reflecting poorly localizable seizures that correspond to recorded clinical seizure events as well as FDG-PET demonstrating decreased uptake in the right anterior and middle temporal lobe (Figure 6.1D) are common findings in HH.

Oral Boards Review—Diagnostic Pearls

1. Gelastic seizures and CPP are the most common presenting symptoms of HH. Hamartomas located anteriorly toward the tuber cinereum are more associated with CPP. Hamartomas located posteriorly toward the mammillary bodies are more associated with seizures.
2. Common diagnostic tests for epilepsy (EEG, FDG-PET, single-photon emission computed tomography [SPECT], and magnetoencephalography [MEG]) often show poorly localized epilepsy in HH and are therefore less useful. Gelastic (laughing) or dacrystic (crying) seizures, even in the presence of other seizure types, should cue physicians to carefully inspect the hypothalamus and surrounding structures on a high-quality MRI scan with thin cuts through the third ventricle and suprasellar/interpeduncular cisterns.
3. Hypothalamic hamartomas are intrinsically epileptogenic. High seizure burden over extended periods of time can lead to secondary epileptogenesis and changes in predominant seizure phenotype over time. Treatment of hamartomas should be performed as early as possible to prevent secondary epileptogenesis, and hamartomas should be treated even when predominant seizure phenotype can be localized to other areas of cortex.
4. The Delalande classification, based on size and location of hamartomas, is a frequently used framework for determining optimal open surgical approaches.

Questions

1. How do these clinical, radiological, and EEG findings influence surgical planning? What surgical options are available for this patient?
2. When should surgery be considered for this patient?
3. What is the Delalande classification?

Decision-Making

In young patients with HH and seizures, aggressive and early surgical treatment of the offending lesion leads to better outcomes. While HH-associated seizures are generally not well controlled with antiepileptic medications, surgical resection/destruction of the hamartoma can halt secondary epileptogenesis as well as progressive behavioral and cognitive decline.

Multiple open surgical approaches can be used to resect HHs, with approach depending on hamartoma size and location. The Delalande classification stratifies HHs into categories based on size and location, and surgical approaches are often discussed using Delalande's stratification. Delalande type 1 HHs are parahypothalamic. They have attachments below the floor of the third ventricle and exist primarily in the suprasellar cistern. Delalande type 1 HHs are classically approached via a pterional transsylvian or subfrontal approach. Orbitozygomatic extension of the craniotomy can be used to minimize brain retraction and allow for improved visualization of the suprasellar region. Delalande type 2 HHs are intrahypothalamic and exist completely above the floor of the third ventricle, within the ventricle. The endoscopic transventricular approach or transcallosal anterior interforniceal approach are typically used for these lesions. The endoscopic transventricular approach has lower morbidity compared to the transcallosal approach, but large lesions and those filling or almost filling the third ventricle are unfavorable through the endoscope. Delalande type 3 HHs are intrahypothalamic and have attachments both above and below the floor of the third ventricle, and type 4 HHs are giant intrahypothalamic lesions. A combination of approaches used to reach above and below the floor of the third ventricle can be employed (e.g., intraventricular endoscopic and orbitozygomatic approach), in a staged manner if necessary, to remove type 3 and 4 HHs.

The open approaches outlined are technically demanding, and as illustrated in several series in the literature, achieving an acceptable rate of morbidity for a surgeon comes only after a significant learning curve. Postoperative seizure freedom rates from open surgery are roughly 50%, with residual seizures stemming from subtotal resection or incomplete disconnection of hamartomatous tissue. Complications of these approaches also reach almost 50% and include hypothyroidism, diabetes insipidus, memory loss, hemiparesis, bradycardia, poikilothermia, visual field deficit, and hyperphagia.

More recently stereotactic radiosurgery (SRS), radio-frequency ablation, and stereotactic laser ablation have been utilized as minimally invasive techniques for HHs. While effects of SRS can take months to become apparent and the amount of tissue ablated with radio-frequency ablation can be imprecise and difficult to monitor directly, laser ablation offers both immediate efficacy and real-time control over ablation volume via MR thermography. Recent series suggested laser ablation of HHs is safer and more effective compared to open surgery. We therefore focus on the technique of MRI-guided stereotactic laser ablation.

Questions

1. What are the main goals of ablating the HH? How can the trajectory of the laser fiber be optimized to address these goals?
2. How can injury to surrounding critical structures be avoided?
3. How is tissue ablation monitored during the procedure?

Surgical Procedure

Laser ablation requires extensive surgical planning and equipment preparation prior to surgery. A single MRI-enabled operating room, or setup to enable sterile drilling and placement of the laser probes with easy transport to obtain an MRI, should be established.

Either of two commercially available laser ablation systems can be utilized for the procedure: the Visualase Thermal Therapy System (Medtronic, Minneapolis, MN) and the Neuroblate Laser Ablation System (Monteris, Plymouth, MN). The Visualase system requires shorter ablation time and has safety measures that allow the user to set maximum temperatures around important anatomical structures; these measures automatically deactivate the laser when the set temperature limit has been reached. The Neuroblate system has one "pick point" function that can be placed near a vital structure to monitor temperature. The Visualase system provides a moderately smaller ablation field compared with the Neuroblate system and may therefore require more trajectories to ablate the same tissue volume. The steps that follow are described for the Visualase system. Thermal energy is delivered via a 10-W, 980-nm diode laser and is controlled with a computer monitoring station. The software for the system uses a model of thermal damage, the Arrhenius equation, to estimate when irreversible cell damage has occurred.

To map the trajectories for ablation, volumetric MRI T1, T2, Fast Imaging Employing Steady-state Acquisition, and gadolinium-enhanced T1 sequences should be acquired. Short-tau inversion recovery (STIR) sequences can be employed to distinguish hypomyelinated fornices and mammillothalamic tracts from the hamartoma. Stereotactic planning software is used to build a three-dimensional representation of the patient's brain and lesion based on these images. The goal of the stereotactic laser ablation is disconnection of the hamartoma from the surrounding tissue in addition to volumetric destruction when feasible. The first target of the ablation should be the inferior, posterior aspect of the hamartoma. On entry into the hamartoma, the trajectory of the laser should be equidistant between the fornix and mammillothalamic tract, as best visualized on T2, STIR, or FIESTA sequences, on the side of the hamartoma that is most anatomically connected. The software then will create an oblique view of the trajectory mapping the trajectory up to the surface of the bone to determine the point of entry in the skull. The Visualase 3-mm diffuser tip can reliably ablate a diameter of up to 14 mm along the trajectory of the laser, occasionally ablating wider depending on the heat sinks encountered. The first trajectory can be planned to allow for disconnection of the hamartoma from the mammillary body, targeting the interface of the lesion and the normal hypothalamic tissue. If the 14-mm expanded trajectory does not include the entire lesion, then a second trajectory should be created to target the remaining area of the lesion. Of note, when mapping the trajectories for ablation, natural heat sinks such as the suprasellar cistern, third ventricle, and foramen of Monro should be appreciated (without direct visualization) and compensated for by planning the trajectory closer to the heat sink. The "probe's eye" view should be used with a T1 gadolinium-infused image sequence to confirm that the planned trajectory is avascular.

Multiple systems, including a frame-based system or frameless stereotactic robot with bone fiducial localization, can be used for implantation of the laser probe. We make a 4-mm stab incision at the entry point for the trajectory and a 3.2-mm burr hole. A 1.9-mm reducing sleeve is used to pass a guide rod through a titanium bone anchor into the burr hole and along the trajectory to the target. The bone anchor is screwed into the skull, and the guide rod is removed. Next, the 1.6-mm laser cannula is advanced along the same tract to the target and a laser fiber with 3 mm diffuser tip is inserted into the cannula. The patient is then placed in the MRI scanner.

A volumetric T1-weighted MR image is acquired to confirm the laser probe trajectory. Oblique MRI cuts are obtained in the plane of the laser trajectory (Figure 6.2A). Temperature limit points are placed near the targeted ablation in critical structures such as the fornices, mammillothalamic tracts, optic chiasm, and interface between the hamartoma and normal hypothalamic tissue. Low-limit markers limit temperatures at a specific point from dropping below 48°C, and high-limit markers limit temperatures to below 90°C. A test dose of laser heat delivery is then performed, at about 8%–12% power, to identify the location of the heat source and adjust the laser diffuser location within the cannula as needed. Laser ablation is then initiated while near real-time MR thermal imaging using fast field echo (FFE) sequences is acquired to monitor the target tissue ablation and surrounding critical structures. An irreversible damage estimate, color coded in orange, then begins to cover the hamartoma. The laser ablation is completed when the entire target is orange.

Postablation imaging with T1-weighted MRI postgadolinium contrast and diffusion-weighted sequences are used to assess the extent of the ablation (Figure 6.2B). The laser fiber and anchor are then removed, and the skin is closed with dissolvable monofilament suture. MR gradient echo or FFE sequences can be acquired to evaluate for hemorrhage.

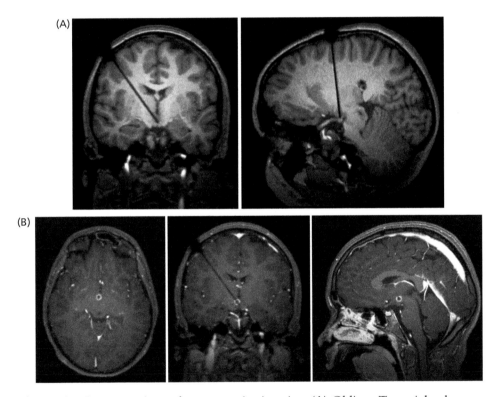

Figure 6.2 Intraoperative and postoperative imaging. (A) Oblique T1-weighted MRI views are generated after insertion of the laser to target. These views allow for subsequent real-time monitoring of ablation volumes via MR thermography. (B) Postablation T1 postcontrast images are obtained after ablation to confirm the ablation volume. The ablated region appears as a hypointense ring-enhancing lesion in the location of the hypothalamic hamartoma.

Oral Boards Review—Management Pearls

1. Hypothalamic hamartomas are notoriously resistant to management with antiepileptics, and medical management trials should not be prolonged.
2. For older, neurologically intact children with a high IQ with minimal seizure burden, SRS should be considered first due to the complication profile of open craniotomy and resection of the HH.
3. Children with high seizure burden and epileptic encephalopathy should undergo stereotactic laser ablation given the complication profile of open craniotomy and unacceptable delay in efficacy of radiosurgery.

Pivot Points

1. In patients with dual pathology and HH, it is tempting but not revealing to pursue invasive monitoring prior to curative surgery because the HH is nearly universally the most epileptogenic lesion in the brain.
2. In strategizing intervention after open surgery, the ablative plan should assess for injury to the fornix/mammillary body/mammillothalamic tract and design the next intervention to avoid contralateral injury in addition to compensating for surgery-induced heat sinks.
3. The HH target can be small and the trajectory length long, making accuracy in stereotaxy crucial and challenging. If the inaccuracy locates the laser source closer to the mammillary body or its connections, then the ablation should be aborted.

Aftercare

Patients are typically admitted one night for observation. There is minimal postoperative wound care for patients undergoing stereotactic laser ablation. Attention after surgery should be focused on preventing postablation edema. We pretreat patients with high-dose oral dexamethasone for 1 week prior to surgery (4 mg every 6 hours) and place patients on a 10-day dexamethasone taper after surgery.

Additionally, serum sodium levels must be closely monitored and corrected following surgery in infants. Disturbances of the supraoptic nucleus or pituitary stalk seen in open or endoscopic HH resections is not seen in stereotactic laser ablation, but infants can exhibit delayed hyponatremia that is easily treated and sometimes prevented by oral sodium supplementation.

Patients should have a follow-up brain MRI with and without contrast at 3 to 6 months to evaluate for completeness of the resection, with repeat follow-up annually thereafter. The neurosurgeon and referring neurologist should evaluate for seizure response to treatment and determine whether the patient is a candidate for re-treatment if the patient has recurrent, incomplete, or no response to the ablation.

Patients with multiple epilepsy phenotypes may experience the "running down phenomenon" after destruction of the HH. During the transition phase of secondary epileptogenesis, when the secondary epileptogenic focus is not yet independent of the primary focus, complete removal of the HH (primary focus) may lead to a gradual decrease and eventual disappearance of the secondary seizure phenotype as the secondary focus fades away. Thus, adequate time between surgery and evaluation for re-treatment (3–9 months) is essential. A transient increase in secondary seizure phenotypes may also occur and resolve with medical management over a similar time period.

Complications and Management

Complications are low in stereotactic laser ablation of HHs compared to the open resection procedures. Complications of stereotactic laser ablation are related to the proximity of critical structures (e.g., mammillary bodies, fornices, pituitary stalk, mammillothalamic tracts) to the planned trajectories and the hypothalamus itself. Diabetes insipidus has occurred rarely, secondary to injury of the nearby pituitary stalk. This can be managed with DDAVP (desmopressin) and follow-up with an endocrinologist. Other endocrine dysfunction, such as hypopituitarism, can be seen and treated with appropriate hormone therapy when diagnosed.

Memory deficits, particularly short-term memory loss, can occur in patients due to closeness of the mammillary bodies to the planned laser trajectory. Injury to the mammillary bodies can be avoided by lowering the low-limit marker used to protect it to 48 and placing it about 2 mm off of the mammillary body border, in the direction of the heat source. Deficits in memory can be difficult to treat and are likely permanent. The patient may require testing accommodations in school and referral to a psychologist to develop techniques and strategies to aid with memory.

Visual changes due to injury of the optic chiasm and optic tracts are very rare after the procedure, likely due to the protection of the optic apparatus in the cistern. Care intraoperatively to set limit points near the targeted ablation in the optic tracts can help prevent this complication.

Last, patients may develop worsening in their nongelastic seizures through a phenomenon of secondary epileptogenesis. Destruction of the primary epileptogenic network through laser ablation of the hamartoma may not destroy other independent networks of epileptogenicity that contribute to a patient's other seizure types. These typically reflect the connectivity of the HH in the mesial temporal lobe and the orbitofrontal lobe. These risks should be discussed with the patient's family prior to surgery, and antiepileptic medication regimens for managing the patient's nongelastic seizures should be developed with the patient's neurologist.

Oral Boards Review—Complications Pearls

1. The most devastating complication in hypothalamic surgery, resective or ablative, is a short-term memory deficit associated with bilateral injury to the mammillary bodies or their outputs, the mammillothalamic tracts, which run near each other superiorly above the mammillary body. All efforts should be taken to avoid any injury, especially bilateral injury.
2. Hypothalamic obesity is rare in laser ablation and can be avoided by ablating only to and not beyond the clearly visible hypothalamus/HH border.

3. The profound cyclic disturbance of sodium control endured in open hypothalamic surgery is not seen in laser ablation, although salt wasting in infants
can be seen. This is easily treated with sodium replacement and occasionally
avoided by perioperative sodium supplementation.

Evidence and Outcomes

There are no prospective randomized controlled trials to compare the efficacy of MRI-
guided stereotactic laser ablation for HHs with more traditional surgeries (e.g., classic
transcallosal approach) or minimally invasive approaches (e.g., endoscopic resection,
radio-frequency thermocoagulation, SRS). The current evidence for stereotactic laser
ablation in these lesions includes several retrospective case series.

- In a series of 14 patients who had HHs and underwent stereotactic laser ablation,
  Wilfong et al. (2013) reported complete seizure freedom in 86% of patients over a
  mean follow-up of 9 months.
- Xu et al. (2018) reviewed the cases of 18 patients who underwent 21 laser interstitial
  thermal therapy treatments for HHs and reported 80% seizure freedom in patients
  with gelastic seizures and 56% seizure freedom in those with nongelastic seizures over
  a mean follow-up 17.4 months.
- In a recent case series of 71 patients (Curry et al. 2018) with a diagnosis of gelastic
  seizures related to HHs treated with stereotactic laser ablation, 93% of patients were
  free of gelastic seizures at 1 year, and 21 patients had secondary seizures reduced by
  ablation.

These case series, among others, have shown excellent seizure freedom outcomes with
low morbidity and shorter hospital stays.

References and Further Reading

Curry DJ, Raskin J, Ali I, Wilfong AA. MR-guided laser ablation for the treatment of hypothalamic
    hamartomas. *Epilepsy Res.* 2018 May;142:131–134. doi:10.1016/j.eplepsyres.2018.03.013.
    Epub 2018 Apr 7. https://www.ncbi.nlm.nih.gov/pubmed/29631919

Kameyama S, Murakami H, Masuda H, Sugiyama I. Minimally invasive magnetic reso-
    nance imaging-guided stereotactic radiofrequency thermocoagulation for epilepto-
    genic hypothalamic hamartomas. *Neurosurgery.* 2009 Sep;65(3):438–449. doi:10.1227/
    01.NEU.0000348292.39252.B5. https://www.ncbi.nlm.nih.gov/pubmed/19687687

Kameyama S, Shirozu H, Masuda H, Ito Y, Sonoda M, Akazawa K. MRI-guided stereotactic
    radiofrequency thermocoagulation for 100 hypothalamic hamartomas. *J Neurosurg.* 2016
    May;124(5):1503–1512. doi:10.3171/2015.4.JNS1582. Epub 2015 Nov 20. https://www.
    ncbi.nlm.nih.gov/pubmed/26587652

Kerrigan JF, Parsons A, Tsang C, Simeone K, Coons S, Wu J. Hypothalamic hamartoma: neuropa-
    thology and epileptogenesis. *Epilepsia.* 2017 Jun;58(Suppl 2):22–31. doi:10.1111/epi.13752.
    https://www.ncbi.nlm.nih.gov/pubmed/28591478

Mittal S, Mittal M, Montes JL, Farmer JP, Andermann F. Hypothalamic hamartomas. Part 1. Clinical, neuroimaging, and neurophysiological characteristics. *Neurosurg Focus*. 2013 Jun;34(6):E6. doi:10.3171/2013.3.FOCUS1355. https://www.ncbi.nlm.nih.gov/pubmed/23724840

Mittal S, Mittal M, Montes JL, Farmer JP, Andermann F. Hypothalamic hamartomas. Part 2. Surgical considerations and outcome. *Neurosurg Focus*. 2013 Jun;34(6):E7. doi:10.3171/2013.3.FOCUS1356. https://www.ncbi.nlm.nih.gov/pubmed/23724841

Wait SD, Abla AA, Killroy BD, Nakaji P, Rekate HL. Surgical approaches to hypothalamic hamartomas. *Neurosurg Focus*. 2011 Feb;30(2):E2. https://www.ncbi.nlm.nih.gov/pubmed/21374830

Wilfong AA, Curry DJ. Hypothalamic hamartomas: optimal approach to clinical evaluation and diagnosis. *Epilepsia*. 2013 Dec;54(Suppl 9):109–114. doi:10.1111/epi.12454. https://www.ncbi.nlm.nih.gov/pubmed/24328883

Xu DS, Chen T, Hlubek RJ, et al. Magnetic resonance imaging-guided laser interstitial thermal therapy for the treatment of hypothalamic hamartomas: a retrospective review. *Neurosurgery*. 2018 Dec 1;83(5):1183–1192. doi:10.1093/neuros/nyx604. https://www.ncbi.nlm.nih.gov/pubmed/29346599

Hippocampal Sclerosis

Zoe E. Teton and Ahmed M. Raslan

Case Presentation

A 37-year-old female first developed seizures with a significant catamenial component at age 23 years while pregnant with a second child. Seizures were described as usually beginning with an aura of déjà vu, before progressing to partial seizures involving visual changes in right visual field, an inability to talk, and cramping/stiffening in the right arm. Often, symptoms will generalize. Seizures occur with ovulation, between days 9 and 16 of menstrual cycle, and happen every month, either once or in clusters. The patient has presented to an emergency department frequently for prolonged seizures requiring administration of intravenous benzodiazepines. The patient has been on multiple antiepileptic drugs (AEDs), including Depakote, topiramate, carbatrol, and Keppra (up to three drugs at a time), and has tried various hormonal birth control options; seizure freedom has not been achieved.

Past electroencephalography (EEG) demonstrated left temporal abnormalities; magnetic resonance imaging (MRI) showed evidence of left mesial temporal sclerosis, and neuropsychologic data suggest a relative deficit of verbal memory compared to visuospatial memory. A phase I video-EEG stay in an epilepsy monitoring unit (EMU) revealed frequent well-formed left frontotemporal spikes (F7/T3/Fp1) and occasional left frontotemporal slowing, with four total seizures captured.

Questions

1. What is the likely diagnosis and appropriate surgical intervention?
2. What are the components of a comprehensive seizure workup prior to consideration for epilepsy surgery?
3. What are possible epilepsy surgery modalities available at modern epilepsy centers?

Assessment and Planning

This patient has undergone a thorough preoperative epilepsy workup and seizure onset localization with phase I (noninvasive video-EEG inpatient) monitoring. At a minimum, all patients should receive a thorough neurologic examination, interictal EEG evaluation, high-resolution epilepsy protocol brain MRI, and a neuropsychologic evaluation as part of the presurgical evaluation. Based on the available data, this patient has nonlesional, focal epilepsy with left mesial temporal lobe onset. Prior to considering any definitive epilepsy surgery, it is critical to complete full seizure-onset localization, as well as comprehensive review of the case with a multidisciplinary conference or committee to achieve consensus among neurologist, neurosurgeon, and patient regarding the most appropriate tailored surgical intervention. In this case, given the focal left temporal onset, the MRI finding of left mesial temporal sclerosis, the consistent semiology, and the neuropsychologic assessment confirming left medial temporal lobe dysfunction (verbal memory), consensus was that this patient was suffering from mesial temporal lobe epilepsy (MTLE), and that selective amygdalohippocampectomy (SAHC) would be the most appropriate treatment.

Questions

1. If the seizure-onset zone was not obvious after phase I monitoring, what would be the most appropriate next step in the workup of this patient?
2. If this patient was not a candidate for open resective surgery, what are the minimally invasive treatment options that could be used for treatment?

Oral Boards Review—Diagnostic Pearls

1. Concordance must be achieved between seizure semiology, imaging findings, and video-EEG evaluation of epileptiform activity prior to proceeding with definitive epilepsy treatment surgery.
2. A full preoperative epilepsy workup includes the components mentioned in addition to a neuropsychiatric evaluation and, at times, an intracarotid sodium amobarbital procedure or Wada test. The Wada test is used to determine if the contralateral temporal lobe is independently able to support memory functions. If concordance of data is not achieved or the seizure-onset zone is still undetermined, phase II monitoring or intracranial video-EEG via subdural surface electrodes or stereoelectroencephalography (sEEG) via depth electrodes may be necessary.
3. Though open resective surgeries remain the most effective surgical treatment for mesial temporal sclerosis and most temporal lobe epilepsy (TLE), newer, more minimally invasive, treatment paradigms include laser interstitial thermal therapy (LITT) and responsive neurostimulation (RNS).

Decision-Making

There are now four standard surgical epilepsy treatments available to patients. Vagal nerve stimulation (VNS) can be an option in medically refractory patients who are not resective surgery candidates. However, VNS is most effective in treating absence-type seizures, while meaningful reduction in other types of epilepsy is more elusive. About a quarter to a half of all patients will experience a 50% reduction in their seizures using VNS.[1–3] RNS is a targeted, neuromodulatory option that is good for treating patients with bilateral seizure onset. RNS leads can be placed in both temporal lobes and use continuous electrocorticography (ECoG) recordings to inform stimulation-mediated treatment of seizures arising from either location. These are both reversible, nonresective treatments that avoid the potential neurocognitive outcomes of permanent resective or ablative treatments and may actually improve cognition as seizures are controlled over time. Notably, however, they are both palliative treatments, and only very rarely do they achieve complete or near-complete seizure freedom.

However, in this case, there was a clear single seizure foci in a location that is safe to resect with minimal cognitive risks. Therefore, resective (anterior temporal lobectomy [ATL], SAHC) or ablative (laser interstitial thermal SAHC) treatments are preferred as these procedures achieve the highest likelihood of seizure freedom. In this particular instance, the complete localization of structural and physiologic pathology to the medial temporal lobe rendered SAHC the preferred option as opposed to the more aggressive option of the ATL. Mounting evidence around the negative cognitive effects associated with long-term use of AEDs and the superiority of surgical outcomes when compared with medical treatment alone has contributed to a paradigm shift in the field toward earlier consideration of resective surgery for patients with MTLE.[4]

Questions

1. What is the most commonly utilized surgical approach in SAHC?
2. What are the available navigation and stereotaxy techniques to ensure accurate target planning in this patient?
3. What is the optimal patient positioning for this procedure?
4. What are the major complications associated with this procedure?

Surgical Procedure

The most commonly utilized surgical approach[5,6] in SAHC, and the one described here, is a transcortical approach via the middle temporal gyrus. Alternative approaches include transsylvian and subtemporal. Stereotactic navigation is utilized to guide this approach. The initial target during the planning phase should be the temporal horn. Registration of the entry point into the sulcus with confirmation of a less than 3-cm distance from the temporal tip is especially important in dominant hemisphere surgery. MRI with placement of fiducial markers is performed just prior to the operation.

The procedure itself is performed in the operating room under routine general anesthesia with endotracheal intubation. Correct positioning is critical in these cases as it allows for direct visualization of the posterior portion of the hippocampus while maintaining a safe trajectory for the entire approach. The patient may be supine or lateral; key to the approach is patient head positioning, which should be strictly lateral where the temple is flat and parallel to the floor. Scalp fiducials are registered, and the planned entry point is marked on the scalp. The head is then shaved, prepped, and draped in standard fashion, and prophylactic antibiotics are given prior to incision. The incision does not need to extend above the superior temporal line, but it is important that it extends inferior enough to ensure adequate exposure, usually just above the zygoma. Craniotomy is performed near the root of the zygoma, and the dura is opened and flapped inferiorly to expose the middle temporal gyrus.

Neuronavigation is then used to locate the area of the cortical incision 2.5–3 cm behind the tip of the temporal lobe, taking care to avoid blood vessels. A 2- to 3-cm corticotomy is

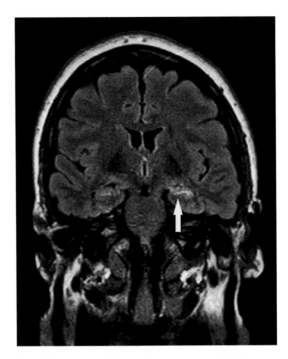

Figure 7.1 Coronal fluid attenuated inversion recovery MRI sequence with suggestion of left hippocampal sclerosis (white arrow).

performed running parallel to the superior temporal sulcus. Dissection is then carried out under microscopic magnification until the temporal horn of the lateral ventricle is entered. Two retractors can be used at this time to maintain optimal visualization. Identification of landmarks prior to surgical resection is critical to this procedure, and the amygdala, the choroid plexus, the hippocampus (Figure 7.1), and the choroidal fissure should all be visualized on the medial inferior walls of the ventricle. A subpial resection of the hippocampus and parahippocampal gyrus is then performed using both microdissection and ultrasonic aspiration. Preservation of the hippocampal sulcus allows for preservation of the hippocampal vessels, which is protective of the anterior choroidal artery. Care should be taken not to violate the pia to preserve the critical structures that lie just beneath it. The dissection should not be carried out superior to the choroidal fissure. Neuronavigation is used to confirm complete resection. The wound is then copiously irrigated and closed (Figure 7.2).

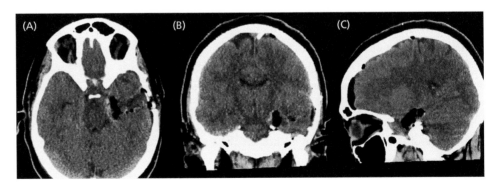

Figure 7.2 Postoperative CT scan without contrast demonstrating resection cavity in (A) axial, (B) coronal, and (C) sagittal planes.

Oral Boards Review—Management Pearls

1. The choroid plexus and the temporal horn can be used as landmarks to maintain orientation of exposure. The resection should remain inferior to the plane of the choroid plexus at all times. Location of the temporal horn should be checked with neuronavigation throughout the procedure: If the stealth is off, the temporal horn usually lies 3 cm deep to the surface of the middle temporal gyrus.
2. When the surgical approach is feeling restricted, a small corticectomy of the inferior temporal gyrus can ease the initial portion of the approach.

Pivot Points

1. An alternative, less invasive, treatment option for this patient would be an ablative treatment such as amygdalohippocampotomy via LITT. Laser ablation is showing promise, but still provides slightly inferior seizure freedom outcome. There might be a benefit from laser ablation in patients with dominant hemisphere TLE given the potential for fewer cognitive side effects[7] (Figure 7.3).
2. If the patient's video–EEG evaluation demonstrated neocortical foci in the temporal lobe, an SAHC would not be appropriate, and a standard open ATL would be required instead.
3. Generally, if intracranial video–EEG evaluation identifies two or more clear epileptogenic zones, this may preclude treatment with SAHC. However, ablative or resective surgeries may help eliminate zones if not located in eloquent cortex and can be paired with RNS as an overall treatment strategy. VNS is an additional surgical option in patients with nonlocalizable seizure onsets and may help decrease seizure frequency and severity.

Aftercare

A postoperative neurological examination should be administered, and head computed tomography (CT) should be performed. AEDs should be resumed immediately following surgery, and the patient should be admitted to the neurological intensive care unit overnight for close neuromonitoring. Typically, the patient will remain in the hospital for 3–4 days before being discharged home.

Complications and Management

The most common issue with SAHC is an incomplete resection. The posterior extent of the resection can be determined by identifying the coronal plane of the collicular plate. Trajectory is important, and inadequate exposure, especially anteriorly and inferiorly can lead to dangerous trajectory shifts posteriorly and superiorly. This can unnecessarily expose and cause potential injury to the sylvian fissure, various language areas, and the optic radiations. Injury to the anterior choroidal artery may lead to temporary or

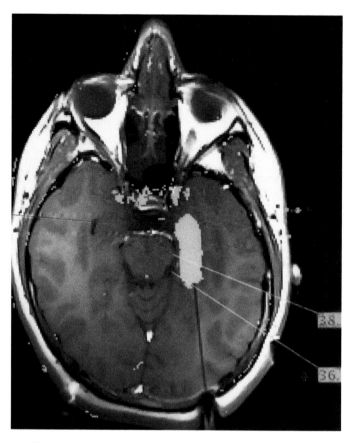

Figure 7.3 Axial T1 contrast with superimposed estimated tissue damage during laser thermal ablation of the left temporal lobe.

permanent neurological deficit. This can be avoided by remaining within the endopial surface at all times. Last, frequent checks with neuronavigation should be employed to avoid injury to the cerebral peduncle.

Oral Boards Review—Complications Pearls

1. By far the most common complications of any temporal lobe surgery are visual field deficits, with incidence up to 100% in ATL surgeries. This is because Meyer's loop travels through the roof and lateral wall of the temporal horn of the lateral ventricle. Selective procedures tend to have lower rates, anywhere from 36% to 53% of cases, and those reported tend to be less severe. These outcomes are purportedly even lower with the subtemporal approach.[5]

2. Ischemia can also occur as a result of SAHC, though the rate of ischemic changes far exceeds that of resultant symptoms. One report noted ischemic changes in nearly half of all SAHC patients, though none demonstrated clinical symptoms from these infarcts.[8] Follow-up neuropsychological study of these patients did demonstrate that verbal memory performance suffered when those infarcts occurred in the language-dominant hemisphere, though verbal fluency and speech comprehension remained largely unaffected.[5]

Evidence and Outcomes

Temporal lobe epilepsy is the most common form of adult localization-related epilepsy, and 80% of these cases originate in the hippocampus.[9] Hippocampal sclerosis (HS) is the single most common cause of medically refractory epilepsy that is also amenable to surgery.[9,10] HS is a combination of astrogliosis and atrophy throughout the hippocampus and is both a cause and a result of seizures originating in this region. It is also among the least likely seizure disorders to be cured by medical treatment alone.[5,10]

A landmark randomized controlled study published by Wiebe et al. in the *New England Journal of Medicine* in 2001 demonstrated that ATL was significantly more effective in preventing awareness-impairing seizures at 1 year of follow-up (58% seizure freedom vs. 8% seizure freedom).[4] Despite this, only 20% of medically refractory patients are referred to a comprehensive epilepsy care center,[11] and only 1.5% of all surgical candidates undergo surgery each year.[12] Neurosurgical treatment of epilepsy has advanced significantly since that initial landmark study and now encompasses a wide array of resective, ablative, and neuromodulatory therapies.

For the treatment of unilateral temporal lobe onset epilepsy, ATL remains the gold standard in terms of achieving seizure control. However, this procedure is associated with significant cognitive deficits including working memory deficits and visual field deficits in up to 100% of cases.[13,14] However, animal models of TLE consistently demonstrated the mesial temporal lobe as being critical to the temporal lobe's epileptogenicity. Thus, the SAHC was explored as an operative option that would provide the same amount of seizure control while preserving the lateral neocortex, temporal pole, and temporal white matter tracts, thus theoretically reducing neuropsychological side effects and morbitity.[5,6] Progress in stereotactic navigation has made SAHC a safer, more accessible, alternative to ATL with comparable seizure-free outcomes.[6] Though the most important outcome after SAHC is the determination of seizure freedom, there have been no randomized controlled trials to date comparing SAHC with medical management. Unfortunately, rates of seizure freedom following ATL are frequently compared with those following SAHC. There have been two large, prospective, randomized clinical trials comparing temporal lobe surgery to medical management in the treatment of MTLE that noted 58%–73% of patients obtained seizure freedom in the surgical group compared with just 0%–8% of patients in the medical management group.

While seizure freedom is of the utmost importance to patients, this benefit can be completely negated if the surgery leads to a significant loss of function. Gleissner et al. reported extensively on cognitive outcomes in 140 patients following SAHC, first after 3 months and then again after 1 year.[15,16] They found that nearly half of the patients experienced some amount of cognitive decline at the 3-month time point, and that this did not improve when they followed up 115 patients after 1 year. They did note that the number one predictor of postoperative performance was preoperative performance. Deficits in verbal memory were most common, though the effect was less pronounced for those who had surgery on the right side.

References and Further Reading

1. A randomized controlled trial of chronic vagus nerve stimulation for treatment of medically intractable seizures. The Vagus Nerve Stimulation Study Group. *Neurology* 1995;45:224–230.

2. Ben-Menachem E, Hellstrom K, Waldton C, Augustinsson LE. Evaluation of refractory epilepsy treated with vagus nerve stimulation for up to 5 years. *Neurology* 1999;52:1265–1267.

3. Ben-Menachem E, Revesz D, Simon BJ, Silberstein S. Surgically implanted and non-invasive vagus nerve stimulation: a review of efficacy, safety and tolerability. *European Journal of Neurology* 2015;22:1260–1268.

4. Wiebe S, Blume WT, Girvin JP, et al. A randomized, controlled trial of surgery for temporal-lobe epilepsy. *The New England Journal of Medicine* 2001;345:311–318.

5. Hoyt AT, Smith KA. Selective amygdalohippocampectomy. *Neurosurgery Clinics of North America* 2016;27:1–17.

6. Spencer D, Burchiel K. Selective amygdalohippocampectomy *Journal of Epilepsy Research and Treatment* 2012;2012:8.

7. Kang JY, Wu C, Tracey J, et al. Laser interstitial thermal therapy for medically intractable mesial temporal lobe epilepsy. *Epilepsia* 2016;57:325–334.

8. Martens T, Merkel M, Holst B, et al. Vascular events after transsylvian selective amygdalohippocampectomy and impact on epilepsy outcome. *Epilepsia* 2014;55:763–769.

9. Tatum W. Mesial temporal lobe epilepsy. *Journal of Clinical Neurophysiology* 2012;29:356–365.

10. Mathon B, Bedos Ulvin L, Adam C, et al. Surgical treatment for mesial temporal lobe epilepsy associated with hippocampal sclerosis. *Revue Neurologique* 2015;171:315–325.

11. Labiner DM, Bagic AI, Herman ST, et al. Essential services, personnel, and facilities in specialized epilepsy centers—revised 2010 guidelines. *Epilepsia* 2010;51:2322–2333.

12. Englot DJ, Ouyang D, Garcia PA, Barbaro NM, Chang EF. Epilepsy surgery trends in the United States, 1990–2008. *Neurology* 2012;78:1200–1206.

13. Ives-Deliperi VL, Butler JT. Naming outcomes of anterior temporal lobectomy in epilepsy patients: a systematic review of the literature. *Epilepsy & Behavior* 2012;24:194–198.

14. Potter JL, Schefft BK, Beebe DW, et al. Presurgical neuropsychological testing predicts cognitive and seizure outcomes after anterior temporal lobectomy. *Epilepsy & Behavior* 2009;16:246–253.

15. Gleissner U, Helmstaedter C, Schramm J, Elger CE. Memory outcome after selective amygdalohippocampectomy in patients with temporal lobe epilepsy: one-year follow-up. *Epilepsia* 2004;45:960–962.

16. Gleissner U, Helmstaedter C, Schramm J, Elger CE. Memory outcome after selective amygdalohippocampectomy: a study in 140 patients with temporal lobe epilepsy. *Epilepsia* 2002;43:87–95.

Neocortical Epilepsy

Zoe E. Teton and Ahmed M. Raslan

Case Presentation

A 28-year-old, right-handed female who has suffered from focal epilepsy since age 11 years is presented. Seizures consist of an aura of "sirens" and a sense of "hyperawareness" with or without progression to oral automatisms, staring, and severe "déjà vu" and are sometimes triggered by music. Occasionally, seizures progress to generalized tonic-clonic (GTC) seizures. Seizures have been consistently refractory to medication, and the patient is unable to tolerate Lamictal and Zonegran due to side effects. Current treatment is with Trileptal and Keppra; however, there are breakthrough seizures (up to 18 per month).

Four years previous, the patient underwent a 2-day epilepsy monitoring unit (EMU) admission that captured right anterior temporal lobe sharp waves on electroencephalogram (EEG), but no seizures. Three years later, a 5-day EMU admission captured three typical focal seizures that originated in the right temporal lobe, with frequent interictal right anterior temporal sharp waves. The patient then underwent 3T epilepsy protocol magnetic resonance imaging (MRI), as well as an experimental 7T MRI protocol; both revealed no lesion. Interictal positron emission tomographic (PET) evaluation was positive for moderately decreased uptake in the anterior and mesial aspects of the temporal lobe, with the right decreased to a greater extent than the left. Subtraction single-photon emission computed tomography (SPECT) demonstrated one GTC seizure of likely right temporal onset and interictal right temporal sharp waves (Figure 8.1).

At a multidisciplinary epilepsy case conference review, consensus was reached that this patient would be a good surgical candidate. However, given several potential right hemispheric foci, the recommendation was made to undergo stereo-EEG (SEEG) with depth electrodes covering the right temporal lobe (mesial structures), Heschel's gyrus, insula, anterior cingulate cortex, and the posterior cingulate cortex. A subsequent 8-day video-EEG monitoring record demonstrated most seizures emanating from the right mesial temporal region with rapid insular engagement. The EEG also noted frequent, rhythmic delta activity in the entorhinal lead within the anterior inferior temporal lobe.

Questions

1. What is the likely diagnosis and appropriate surgical intervention?
2. What are the components of a comprehensive seizure workup prior to consideration for epilepsy surgery?
3. What are the possible epilepsy surgery modalities available at modern epilepsy centers?

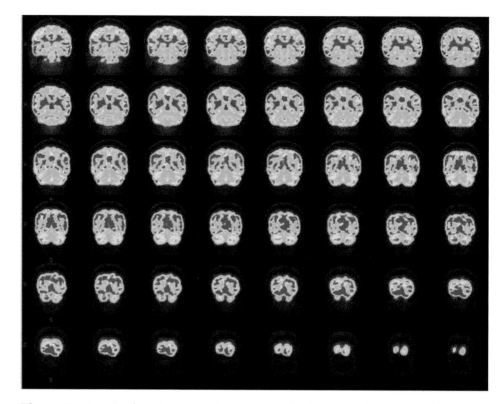

Figure 8.1 Interictal positron emission tomography demonstrating moderately decreased uptake in the anterior and mesial aspects of the temporal lobes, with the right decreased to a greater extent than the left.

Assessment and Planning

This is a classic case of the so-called imaging-normal temporal/limbic lobe epilepsy. In addition, the ictal EEG and semiology did not demonstrate a clear ictal onset zone. The borderline positive SPECT examination suggests a right temporal lobe onset, but it is not independently sufficient to warrant the decision to proceed with respective surgery. Therefore, a phase II monitoring with SEEG was indicated. The SEEG coverage for this case was the right temporal lobe in addition to the insula, anterior cingulate gyrus, posterior cingulate gyrus, and the orbitofrontal cortex (Figure 8.2). Ictal EEG with intracranial electrodes implanted revealed simultaneous onset of seizures from both medial and neocortical temporal lobe with spread to insular and cingulate electrodes. The musicogenic feature of seizure triggering in her semiology was an indicator of potential neocortical onset near Heschel's gyrus.

Patient neuropsychological assessment confirmed nondominant hemisphere dysfunction. This, together with right-sided SPECT/PET lateralization, semiology, and phase II monitoring data, pointed—with a high degree of confidence—to right temporal lobe onset epilepsy.

In this case, given the neocortical seizure onsets, consensus was reached that right anterior temporal lobectomy (ATL) would give the patient the best chance of seizure cure.

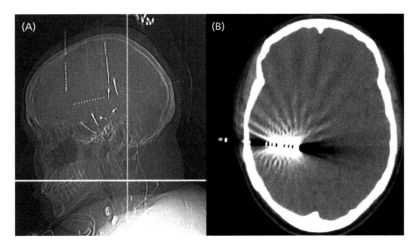

Figure 8.2 Stereo-EEG imaging. (A) Sagittal x-ray demonstrating multiple right hemispheric depth electrodes targeting the mesial temporal lobe, Heschel's gyrus, the insula, the anterior cingulate cortex, and the posterior cingulate cortex. (B) Axial noncontrast CT scan demonstrating SEEG depth electrode targeting right temporal lobe mesial structures.

Questions

1. If phase II evaluation had localized seizures to the mesial temporal lobe exclusively, what would have been the most appropriate surgical intervention?
2. If phase II evaluation had demonstrated bitemporal seizure onset, what minimally invasive treatment options would have been recommended?

Oral Boards Review—Diagnostic Pearls

1. Concordance must be achieved between seizure semiology, imaging findings, and video-EEG evaluation of epileptiform activity prior to proceeding with definitive epilepsy treatment surgery.
2. A full preoperative epilepsy workup includes the components mentioned, as well as neuropsychiatric evaluation, intracarotid sodium amobarbital procedure or Wada test, and intracranial video-EEG via subdural surface electrodes or SEEG via depth electrodes if necessary.
3. Though open resective surgeries remain the most effective surgical treatment for mesial temporal sclerosis and most temporal lobe epilepsy (TLE), newer, more minimally invasive treatment paradigms include laser interstitial thermal therapy (LITT) and responsive neurostimulation (RNS).

Decision-Making

There are a number of minimally invasive treatment options for medically intractable epilepsy patients who are not considered surgical candidates. Both vagal nerve stimulation

(VNS) and RNS are reversible, nonresective treatments that avoid the potential negative neurocognitive outcomes sometimes associated with the permanent respective or ablative treatments and may improve cognition as seizure control is maintained over time. VNS is most effective at treating absence seizures, though efficacy in reducing the seizure rate by even 50% ranges anywhere from 24% to 48% of patients. RNS is a targeted treatment option that is especially helpful in patients with bilateral onset as leads can be placed in both temporal lobes.

While these options are certainly desirable in a certain subset of patients, resective surgery has the highest likelihood of achieving seizure freedom and is the preferred treatment for patients with a clear, single, seizure focus that is safe to resect with minimal cognitive risks. In this case, had the patient's seizures originated in the mesial temporal lobe only, she would have been a candidate for selective amygdalohippocampectomy (SAHC) or an ablative treatment such as laser interstitial thermal SAHC. ATL has virtually identical therapeutic efficacy as SAHC with marginally higher rates of postoperative neurocognitive deficit. Both have demonstrated exemplary rates of seizure freedom as compared with medical treatment alone.

Patients with normal imaging but SPECT/PET positive imaging are candidates for ATL, as was the case here. However, the decision was made to proceed with SEEG because of the multiple semiologies and the musicogenic aspect of her seizures. Understanding the exact cortical onset was important as preservation of Heschel's gyrus is a concern in this case.

Questions

1. What is the anatomical landmark for the posterior extent of hippocampal resection?
2. What resection length should you aim for in the dominant temporal lobe versus the nondominant temporal lobe?
3. What are the major complications associated with this procedure?

Surgical Procedure

The traditional surgical approach[1,2] to the ATL should consist of three main components: temporal craniotomy, removal of the neocortical block, followed by removal of the mesial temporal structures. The patient should be placed in three-point head fixation with the maxilla pointing directly upward and the head at 90°. Incision should be made anterior to the tragus and below the zygoma, following a curvilinear or question mark shape to just above the superior temporal line. Temporalis and temporalis fascia are then elevated from the skull and reflected outward. The craniotomy should extend slightly above the squamousal suture with burr holes placed on the frontal side of the sphenoid wing (near the "keyhole") and on the temporal squama just above the root of the zygoma.

The resection technique begins with lateral neocortical resection, followed by exposure within the temporal horn and resection of the amygdala and uncus. At this point, the hippocampus and the parahippocampus are isolated. These can be mobilized from anterior to posterior and resected en bloc; alternatively, the hippocampus and

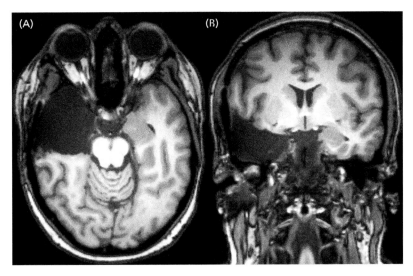

Figure 8.3 Postoperative MRI sequences demonstrating (A) axial and (B) coronal views of the resection cavity for the right anterior temporal lobectomy.

parahippocampal areas are removed using ultrasonic aspiration in situ via an endopial approach. Small hippocampal arteries and veins residing in the hippocampal mesentery should be coagulated and cut at their most distal point to avoid coagulation of an intra-arachnoid loop of the anterior choroidal artery. The anatomical landmark for the posterior extent of the resection is the collicular plate. The resection length should be measured from the greater wing of the sphenoid to what remains of the middle temporal gyrus and should be 2–2.5 cm in the dominant temporal lobe and 4–4.5 cm in the nondominant lobe. The surgical field is then copiously irrigated and closed in standard multilayer fashion (Figure 8.3).

Oral Boards Review—Management Pearls

1. The operating surgeon should take care to preserve the vein of Labbé as well as the prominent temporobasilar veins.[2]
2. Both the temporal horn and tentorial dura are important landmarks to visualize to prevent blind dissection too far medially. The temporomesial pia should be preserved as a protective layer over the underlying critical neurovascular structures.

Alternative Management Strategies

1. If intracranial video-EEG evaluation reveals a clear unilateral mesial temporal lobe onset, it may also be reasonable to proceed with an ablative treatment such as AHC via LITT or SAHC.
2. If SEEG evaluation were to reveal bilateral temporal lobe onset, it may be reasonable to consider a more minimally invasive treatment option such as RNS or VNS. Both of these treatments have been shown to help decrease seizure frequency and severity.

If greater than two clear epileptogenic zones are identified, these treatments may be combined—ablative or resective surgery to eliminate zones not in eloquent cortex and then subsequent pairing with RNS or VNS for a more comprehensive treatment strategy.

Aftercare

A postoperative neurological examination should be administered and head computed tomography (CT) performed. Antiepileptic drugs can be resumed immediately following surgery, and the patient should be admitted to the neurological intensive care unit overnight for close neuromonitoring. Typically, the patient will remain in the hospital for 3–4 days before being discharged home. Antiepileptic medications should be continued both pre- and postoperatively. These medications can be tapered after 3–12 months of seizure freedom.

Complications and Management

Mortality is low in these cases and is observed less than 1% of the time. Morbidity is higher, around 5%, but only 1%–2% of these instances are permanent. The most common complication is visual field defects, and they are observed in up to 50% of patients.[2] This is in addition to the nearly universal side effect of upper contralateral quadrantanopia. Neuropsychological performance can deteriorate in up to 50% of patients, resulting in cognitive and memory decline, especially in dominant lobe procedures. On the other hand, neuropsychological performance will improve in up to one-third of cases if seizure freedom is attained.

Oral Boards Review—Complications Pearls

1. While neuronavigation can certainly be used to avoid dissection into the basal ganglia while resecting the amygdala, this continues to be a procedure that relies heavily on anatomical landmarks to guide resection. It is important to visualize the temporal horn and tentorial dura to avoid dissection too medially.
2. The temporomesial pia arachnoid should be preserved to avoid the neurovascular structures that lie underneath. As these are approached, the ultrasonic aspirator should be turned down. In the event of bleeding, apply sponge or fibrillary hemostatics and avoid coagulation whenever possible.
3. The length of resection should stay within 4–4.5 cm in the dominant lobe and between 5 and 5.5 cm in the nondominant lobe. A functional MRI should be ordered if there is any question of lobar dominance.

Evidence and Outcomes

Temporal lobe epilepsy is the most common form of adult localization-related epilepsy.[3] While 80% of patients are shown to have mesial temporal seizure onset, neocortical TLE encompasses a broader group of epilepsies generally characterized by an aura (somato-sensory or psychic/déjà vu similar to the case presented here), followed by contralateral clonic activity that will very often generalize.[4] Of patients with this disease, up to 30% will remain refractory to medication. Medically refractory epilepsy has come to be defined as a failure of two separate antiepileptic drugs, whether they are administered sequentially as a monotherapy or as a combined course.[2] The superiority of surgery in these patients was ultimately established in 2001 by a landmark randomized controlled trial conducted by Wiebe et al. The trial demonstrated an obvious benefit to surgery over medication in the treatment of patients at 1-year follow-up, with 58% of the surgical patients remaining seizure free, while just 8% in the medication group remained seizure free.[5] This effect has been consistently demonstrated with 60%–80% of patients with ATL achieving seizure freedom in follow-up studies and in many cases less than 5% of those that pursue medical treatment alone achieving that same effect. ATL continues to be considered the gold standard in achieving seizure freedom but does come with a significant set of cognitive deficits.[6,7] While the Weibe et al. trial examined ATL specifically, the thought gradually emerged that the more targeted SAHC would be able to yield similar rates of seizure freedom while preserving neurocognitive outcomes.[8] In a 2013 meta-analysis, Josephson et al. confirmed that ATL did indeed achieve statistically significantly higher Engel outcome scale class I outcomes than those who underwent SAHC, but noted that this may be at the cost of higher neuropsychological deficit.[9] This meta-analysis was unable to determine the degree of difference within neurocognitive outcomes due to heterogeneity in reporting paradigms, but the study does underscore the importance of accurately identifying the seizure-onset zone (SOZ) when completing an epilepsy workup in this patient population. Surgical complication rates of death or serious neurological disability were comparable between the two procedures; 0%–3.1% in ATL and 0%–2.4% in SAHC.[9]

Initial epilepsy workup should include long-term noninvasive surface EEG monitoring, referred to as a phase I evaluation. In approximately 25% of cases, however, this is not sufficient to determine a SOZ, and in these cases, phase II long-term intracranial monitoring is required.[10] Phase II monitoring may be achieved with subdural strip electrodes but has become increasingly reliant on SEEG.[11,12] A major difference between the two methods is that SEEG allows exploration in three-dimensional space within the brain, and subcortical seizure activity can be recorded. Rather than sampling over contiguous stretches of cortex, SEEG utilizes predetermined and specifically directed areas based on a sound preoperative hypothesis.[13] SEEG has also been lauded as superior to subdural grids as placement is minimally invasive and does not require the large craniotomy required of subdural grid placement and displays relatively low complication rates.[13] SEEG evaluations are conducted to determine (1) the SOZ; (2) the wider epileptic network (this can be defined simply as the brain areas proximal to the SOZ or more broadly may include distal areas, even those contralateral to the SOZ); (3) any eloquent cortex that may border the SOZ; and (4) what constitutes the area of "normal brain" around the SOZ.[13] If the SEEG evaluation identifies the SOZ as involving the lateral neocortex, then SAHC is no longer an option, and the treatment team can definitively move forward with the ATL (as in the case presented here). Complication rates for SEEG are notably lower than those for subdural strip or grid electrodes, with a less than 1% clinically significant hemorrhage rate and an infection rate of less than 4%.[14,15]

References and Further Reading

1. Elliott RE, Bollo RJ, Berliner JL, et al. Anterior temporal lobectomy with amygdalo-hippocampectomy for mesial temporal sclerosis: predictors of long-term seizure control. *Journal of Neurosurgery*. 2013;119(2):261–272.

2. Schaller K, Cabrilo I. Anterior temporal lobectomy. *Acta Neurochirurgica*. 2016;158(1):161–166.

3. Tatum WO 4th. Mesial temporal lobe epilepsy. *Journal of Clinical Neurophysiology: Official Publication of the American Electroencephalographic Society*. 2012;29(5):356–365.

4. Kennedy JD, Schuele SU. Neocortical temporal lobe epilepsy. *Journal of Clinical Neurophysiology: Official Publication of the American Electroencephalographic Society*. 2012;29(5):366–370.

5. Wiebe S, Blume WT, Girvin JP, Eliasziw M. A randomized, controlled trial of surgery for temporal-lobe epilepsy. *The New England Journal of Medicine*. 2001;345(5):311–318.

6. Ives-Deliperi VL, Butler JT. Naming outcomes of anterior temporal lobectomy in epilepsy patients: a systematic review of the literature. *Epilepsy & Behavior*. 2012;24(2):194–198.

7. Potter JL, Schefft BK, Beebe DW, Howe SR, Yeh HS, Privitera MD. Presurgical neuropsychological testing predicts cognitive and seizure outcomes after anterior temporal lobectomy. *Epilepsy & Behavior*. 2009;16(2):246–253.

8. Spencer D, Burchiel K. Selective amygdalohippocampectomy. *Epilepsy Research and Treatment*. 2012;2012:382095.

9. Josephson CB, Dykeman J, Fiest KM, et al. Systematic review and meta-analysis of standard vs. selective temporal lobe epilepsy surgery. *Neurology*. 2013;80(18):1669–1676.

10. Diehl B, Luders HO. Temporal lobe epilepsy: when are invasive recordings needed? *Epilepsia*. 2000;41(Suppl 3):S61–S74.

11. Bancaud J, Angelergues R, Bernouilli C, et al. Functional stereotaxic exploration (SEEG) of epilepsy. *Electroencephalography and Clinical Neurophysiology*. 1970;28(1):85–86.

12. Talairach J, Bancaud J, Bonis A, Szikla G, Tournoux P. Functional stereotaxic exploration of epilepsy. *Confinia Neurologica*. 1962;22:328–331.

13. Kalamangalam GP, Tandon N. Stereo-EEG implantation strategy. *Journal of Clinical Neurophysiology: Official Publication of the American Electroencephalographic Society*. 2016;33(6):483–489.

14. Gonzalez-Martinez J, Mullin J, Vadera S, et al. Stereotactic placement of depth electrodes in medically intractable epilepsy. *Journal of Neurosurgery*. 2014;120(3):639–644.

15. Schmidt RF, Wu C, Lang MJ, et al. Complications of subdural and depth electrodes in 269 patients undergoing 317 procedures for invasive monitoring in epilepsy. *Epilepsia*. 2016;57(10):1697–1708.

Bitemporal Focus Epilepsy

Allen L. Ho and Casey H. Halpern

Case Presentation

The patient is a 28-year-old male who first developed seizures at the age of 17. His seizures are general tonic-clonic seizures that begin with an aura of sparkling lights, nausea, and confusion and progress to nonresponsiveness. These seizures all last less than 5 minutes. He has about one seizure a week, but they sometimes cluster, and the frequency appears to be increasing over time. The patient has been on several antiepileptic drugs (AEDs), including Lamictal, Keppra, and oxcarbazepine and is now maintained primarily on valproic acid, which has controlled the severity, but not the frequency, of his seizures.

At initial evaluation, his magnetic resonance imaging (MRI) demonstrated no frank abnormalities. Interictal fluorodeoxyglucose positron emission tomography (FDG-PET) evaluation was positive for mild hypometabolic activity in the left anterior temporal lobe. He completed a neuropsychiatric evaluation, which was significant for mild impairment of functions subserved by both the left and right temporal regions, with more difficulty on left hemisphere tasks. He had asymmetrically lower performance with his right hand on motor testing. He has completed several routine electroencephalographic (EEG) studies that demonstrated occasional bilateral independent temporal spikes and infrequent left temporal slowing. He underwent a phase I video-EEG stay in the epilepsy monitoring unit (EMU), which revealed intermittent left temporal slowing; frequent sharp spikes over temporal regions (at T1-T3 and at T2-T4); 18 right temporal seizures on eight occasions of possible left-sided onset due to the presence of left temporal sentinel spikes. On review of the patient at a multidisciplinary epilepsy conference, the decision was made to pursue phase II high-density intracranial EEG with placement of bilateral orbitofrontal and anterior and posterior temporal (hippocampal) depth electrodes for localization of the seizure-onset zone. This 3-day phase II evaluation was significant for copious bitemporal spiking, with independent activity in the left posterior hippocampus and in the right anterior hippocampus. The patient also experienced nine simple partial seizures, with six right hippocampal onsets and three left hippocampal onsets. Spiking was approximately 5-fold more prevalent in the left hippocampus, though more seizures emanated from the right.

Questions

1. What are the likely diagnosis and appropriate surgical intervention?
2. What are the components of a comprehensive seizure workup prior to consideration for epilepsy surgery?
3. What are the possible epilepsy surgery modalities available at modern epilepsy centers?

Assessment and Planning

This patient has undergone a thorough preoperative epilepsy workup and examination of seizure onset localization with both phase I (noninvasive video-EEG inpatient study) and phase II (invasive surface or depth electrode video-EEG inpatient study) monitoring (Figure 9.1). Based on the available data, the patient has nonlesional focal epilepsy with bilateral temporal lobe onsets. It is critical prior to considering any definitive epilepsy surgery to complete a full comprehensive seizure-onset localization, as well as full workup and data review with a multidisciplinary conference or committee to achieve consensus among neurologist, neurosurgeon, and patient regarding the most appropriate tailored surgical intervention. In this case, given the bilateral temporal onsets,

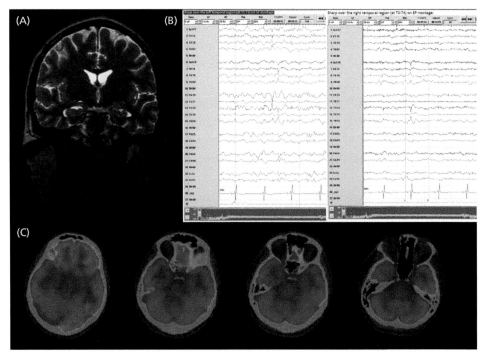

Figure 9.1 Preoperative diagnostic workup. (A) Anatomic MRI evaluation demonstrating normal-appearing hippocampi and temporal lobes bilaterally. (B) Sample from video-EEG evaluation demonstrating interictal activity in the form of broad field sharp spikes over T1–T3 and T2–T4 on the left (left) and sharp spikes over T2–T4 on the right (right). (C) Interictal FDG-PET demonstrating mild hypometabolic activity in the left anterior temporal lobe.

consensus was achieved that responsive neurostimulation (RNS) would be the most appropriate treatment for this patient.

Questions

1. If phase II evaluation had not been available, what would have been the most appropriate surgical intervention?
2. How effective is RNS compared to more ablative therapies?

Oral Boards Review—Diagnostic Pearls

1. Concordance must be achieved between seizure semiology, imaging findings, and video-EEG evaluation of epileptiform activity prior to proceeding with definitive epilepsy treatment surgery.
2. A full preoperative epilepsy workup includes the components mentioned as well as neuropsychiatric evaluation, intracarotid sodium amobarbital procedure or Wada test, and intracranial video-EEG via subdural surface electrodes or stereoelectroencephalography (SEEG) via depth electrodes if necessary.
3. Though open resective surgeries remain the most effective surgical treatment for mesial temporal sclerosis and most temporal lobe epilepsy, newer, more minimally invasive treatment paradigms include laser interstitial thermal therapy (LITT) and RNS.

Decision-Making

There are now four standard surgical epilepsy treatments available to patients. Generally, if there is a clear single seizure focus that is safe to resect with minimal cognitive risks, then resective (anterior temporal lobectomy [ATL], selective amygdalohippocampectomy) or ablative (laser interstitial thermal selective amygdalohippocampotomy) treatments are appropriate in order to achieve the highest likelihood of seizure freedom. However, in this patient, resective and ablative surgical options are not appropriate given the bilateral temporal onsets identified during phase II investigation. Vagal nerve stimulation (VNS) can be an option in medically refractory patients who are not candidates for resective surgery. However, VNS is most effective in treating absence-type seizures, and while in other types of epilepsy seizure severity and frequency can be reduced with VNS, meaningful seizure frequency reduction is elusive. RNS is a targeted, neuromodulatory option that is the best treatment for this patient. Given his bilateral onsets, RNS leads can be placed in both temporal lobes and long-term electrocorticography (ECoG) recordings and stimulation-mediated treatment of seizures arising from both temporal lobes can be achieved. This is a reversible, nonresective treatment that avoids the potential neurocognitive outcomes of permanent resective or ablative treatments and may actually improve cognition as seizure control is achieved over time. This therapy has had demonstrated long-term efficacy in both mesial and nonmesial temporal lobe epilepsy.

Questions

1. What is the optimal RNS lead placement and configuration for this patient?
2. What are the available navigation and stereotaxy techniques to ensure accurate lead placement for this patient?
3. What are the major complications associated with this procedure?

Surgical Procedure

There are several options for RNS lead placement for temporal lobe epilepsy treatment, but the most common configuration involves two longitudinal depth electrodes placed along the long axis of the hippocampus with the distal tip seated in either the amygdala or the hippocampus. Current RNS systems are only able to connect to two electrodes. However, there are numerous configuration options with both depth and strip electrodes for temporal lobe epilepsy, and often additional leads may be placed but left unconnected to be connected in the future or for future RNS upgrades that may accommodate more than two leads. There are also several different options for stereotactic placement of the depth electrode, including frame-based, frameless, and robotic stereotaxy systems. Imaging guidance may be necessary depending on stereotactic technique, and intraoperative computed tomographic (CT) imaging may be helpful for image registration and to confirm electrode placement.

Given the need to perform a craniotomy to fit the RNS device, a frameless system with intraoperative CT registration may be the least cumbersome technique that maintains adequate stereotactic accuracy. Briefly, the patient is brought into the operating room, and general endotracheal anesthesia is administered. The patient is positioned prone with head neutral and rigidly fixed in pins with the neck slightly extended and the head of the bed elevated to allow adequate access to perform a small parietal craniotomy. A reference arc is attached to the head frame, and a volumetric CT scan through the entire cranial vault is carried out with an intraoperative CT scanner. This scan is then autoregistered with the preoperative anatomic MRI scan.

Targets are planned within the image guidance software for the hippocampus bilaterally, and bilateral occipital entry points are identified on the skin. Incisions should be planned so that an adequate craniotomy may be performed to fit the RNS unit template in the parietal region with either a separate incision or ipsilaterally connecting incisions over the occipital entry points of the hippocampal leads. The head is then shaved, prepped, and draped in standard fashion and prophylactic antibiotics given prior to incision.

Generally, both leads are placed prior to completing the craniotomy to implant the RNS unit. A small incision is made over the entry points, and utilizing the Vertek aiming device that has been aligned to trajectory, a small 3-mm burr hole are made. A guide cannula is placed, and the lead is then advanced through the cannula to the target, and the stylet is removed. The lead is adhered to the bone utilizing a small electrode cover, and the same procedure is repeated on the contralateral side.

A parietal incision is then made to seat the stimulator. A craniotomy is fashioned using the template as a guide in order to accommodate the ferrule. The ferrule is secured into place with 4-mm bone screws, and a periosteal is utilized to tunnel the electrode leads to the RNS device, which is then locked into the ferrule tray. Excess lead is coiled within a subcutaneous pocket away from the device. Impedances are confirmed to be normal and ECoG interrogated for expected individual electrode recordings (Figure 9.2). The wound is then copiously irrigated and closed in standard multilayer fashion (Figure 9.3).

Oral Boards Review—Management Pearls

1. One of the main advantages of RNS in treatment of temporal lobe epilepsies is its ability to monitor both hemispheres if there is any question about a bilateral onset. Standard placement should include a depth electrode placed down the long axis of the hippocampus bilaterally. In patients with mesial temporal onsets, for a significant number of patients bilateral RNS will demonstrate a different lateralization of seizures than previous diagnostic testing.

2. A thoughtful approach to RNS placement relative to electrode placement and wiring must be taken given that many of these patients will inevitably undergo a revision operation to replace the RNS unit battery several years down the line. Surgeon preference may favor a C-shaped incision that avoids overlapping any wires or connection points with the device to facilitate access in revision surgeries.

3. For complex cases of seizure localization or multiple onsets, there may be some utility in placing more than two electrodes. This allows for switching of the electrode hookup at the unit itself without the need for large exposure if necessary. Future iterations of the RNS device will enable greater than two electrodes for recording/stimulation, so the decision regarding number of electrodes placed can be made with this in mind.

Pivot Points

1. If intracranial video–EEG evaluation reveals a clear unilateral temporal lobe onset, it may also be reasonable to proceed with an ablative treatment such as amygdalohippocampotomy via LITT, standard open ATL, or selective amygdalohippocampectomy.

2. Generally, if intracranial video–EEG evaluation identified greater than two clear epileptogenic zones, this may preclude treatment with an RNS device. Ablative or resective surgeries may help eliminate zones if not located in eloquent cortex and can be paired with RNS as an overall treatment strategy. VNS is an additional surgical option in patients with nonlocalizable seizure onsets and may help decrease seizure frequency and severity.

Aftercare

Postoperatively, the patient should undergo CT scanning if one was not completed intraoperatively to confirm lead position and rule out any intracranial hemorrhage. The

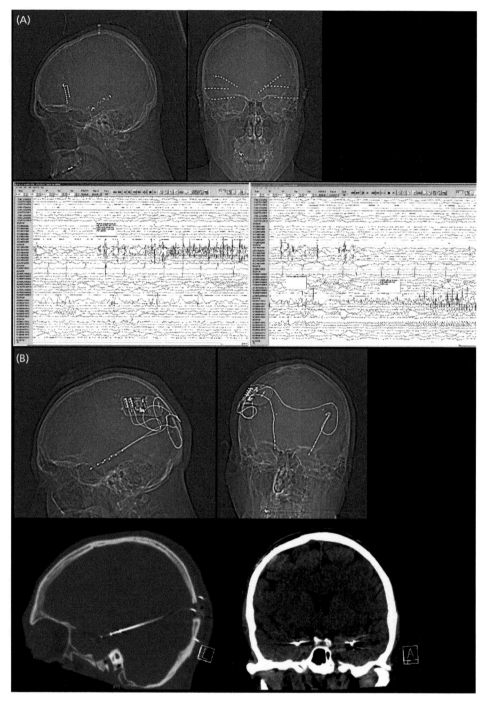

Figure 9.2 Surgical diagnostic evaluation and RNS placement. (A) AP and lateral skull x-ray demonstrating placement of bilateral frontal and temporal stereotactic depth EEG electrodes (top). Sample (left, bottom) from video–depth EEG evaluation demonstrating a simple partial seizure arising from the right hippocampal lead. Sample (right, bottom) from video–depth EEG evaluation demonstrating a simple partial seizure arising from the left hippocampal lead. (B) AP and lateral skull x-ray demonstrating placement of bilateral temporal hippocampal RNS leads (top). Sagittal and coronal noncontract CT scans demonstrating intracranial placement of RNS leads are shown at the bottom.

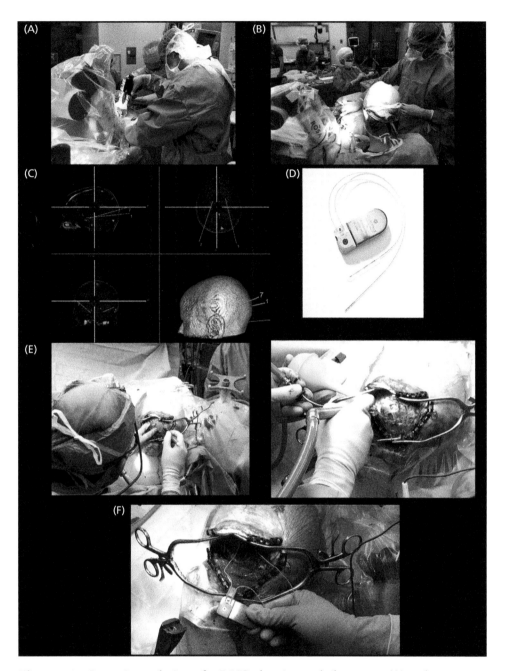

Figure 9.3 Operative technique for RNS planning and placement. (A) and
(B) Utilization of ROSA robot for placement of stereotactic depth EEG electrodes
for intracranial video–depth EEG evaluation. (C) Planning software for placement of
bilateral hippocampal RNS depth electrodes. (D) RNS device with paddle and depth
electrodes. (E) RNS template utilized to plan and complete craniotomy for placement
of ferrule. (F) Attachment of previously placed RNS electrodes to RNS unit prior to
implantation.

patient should then be admitted to either the intensive care unit (ICU) or neurosurgical step-down unit for close neuromonitoring. AEDs should be resumed immediately, and the patient should complete a full 24-hour course of prophylactic antibiotics. After 24 hours of postoperative inpatient care, if the patient is otherwise stable and meets normal criteria for discharge, the patient may be discharged home. Optimal postoperative incision care is critical given the presence of underlying hardware.

Complications and Management

In the initial trial cohort, there was a postoperative intracranial hemorrhage rate of 3%, of which half required surgical evacuation.[1] If there is any evidence of intracranial hemorrhage, the patient should be admitted to the ICU for close neuromonitoring, and interval repeat CT scanning should be completed to ensure stability of the hemorrhage. Epidural or large subdural or intracerebral hemorrhages may require surgical evacuation and possible explantation. In the initial trial cohort, there was a total infection rate of 5%. Half of these infections occurred immediately postoperatively, and half occurred after the postoperative period due to secondarily infected seizure-induced head lacerations. Half of the patients with infections were ultimately explanted.[1] Given the concern for seeding hardware infection, any deep tissue infection that extends beyond the dermal layer should be explored and considered for explantation.

Oral Boards Review—Complications Pearls

1. Trajectory planning for both depth and surface electrode implantation is critical for avoiding an intracranial hemorrhage. This most commonly occurs from surface cortical veins, so dural and cortical entry point selection must be done with this in mind. Utilization of a high-resolution vascular imaging protocol (either CT angiogram, magnetic resonance [MR] angiography, or digital subtraction angiography) merged with a volumetric, anatomic MRI for trajectory planning can help avoid trajectories that involve cortical veins, traversing sulci, or ventricles or larger intraparenchymal vessels that lead to increased intracranial hemorrhage risk.

2. Given the hardware implantation inherent in this procedure, the risks of infection and its sequelae are higher than for most other resective or ablative epilepsy surgeries. Large RNS studies have revealed an infection rate of around 5%, of which half will require explantation. Many of these patients will have had intracranial video-EEG monitoring prior to surgery with external electrodes creating a "clean/contaminated" wound; thus it is generally prudent to wait a period of time (several weeks to months) after completing intracranial monitoring prior to permanent implantation of the RNS device to ensure no intervening wound infection.

Evidence and Outcomes

Over 800,000 Americans continue to experience seizures despite AEDs,[2] and there is a less than 5% rate of seizure control after a patient has failed two prior AEDs.[3] The appropriate management of these medically refractory epilepsy patients is workup at a comprehensive epilepsy center (CEC) for seizure localization and consideration for epilepsy surgery. A landmark randomized controlled study published by Wiebe et al. in the *New England Journal of Medicine* in 2001 demonstrated that ATL was significantly more effective in preventing awareness-impairing seizures at 1 year of follow-up (58% seizure freedom vs. 8% seizure freedom).[4] Despite this, only 20% of medication-refractory patients are being referred to a CEC,[5] and only 1500 of 100,000 surgical candidates undergo surgery each year.[6]

Neurosurgical treatment of epilepsy has advanced significantly since that initial landmark study and now encompasses a wide array of resective, ablative, and neuromodulatory therapies. For the treatment of unilateral temporal lobe onset epilepsy, ATL remains the gold standard in terms of achieving seizure control. However, there are significant cognitive deficits, including working memory deficits, that are seen with this procedure.[7,8] RNS was developed in order to obtain long-term ECoG information from patients with epilepsy, allow for stimulation-driven interruption of seizures prior to onset, and avoid cognitive side effects associated with ablative and resective surgeries.

In 2011, the first multicenter, double-blind, randomized controlled trial of RNS was published. This study demonstrated a significant reduction in seizures in patients treated with RNS versus sham (37.9% reduction with RNS vs. 17.3% with sham, $p = .012$). There were also significant improvements in quality of life and no deterioration in mood or neuropsychological function.[9,10]

Responsive neurostimulation is a dynamic therapy that allows for tailoring of stimulation parameters over time, and at 7-year follow-up, median seizure reduction had steadily improved annually to a rate of 72%.[11] In nonmesial temporal lobe epilepsy patients specifically, median reduction in seizure frequency was 70%, with a 68% responder rate (greater than 50% reduction).[12] In terms of lateralization, in patients with mesial temporal onsets there was a significant number of patients for whom bilateral RNS demonstrated a different lateralization of seizures than previous diagnostic testing. For patients with confirmed unilateral onsets preoperatively, 64% were discovered to have bilateral onsets. For patients with confirmed bilateral onsets preoperatively, 13% only had unilateral onsets. Finally, time to detect bilateral Mesial Temporal Sclerosis (MTS) seizure onsets took longer than 4 weeks in 32% of patients.[13]

References and Further Reading

1. Bergey GK, Morrell MJ, Mizrahi EM, et al. Long-term treatment with responsive brain stimulation in adults with refractory partial seizures. *Neurology.* 2015;84(8):810–817. doi:10.1212/WNL.0000000000001280

2. Hesdorffer DC, Beck V, Begley CE, et al. Research implications of the Institute of Medicine Report, Epilepsy Across the Spectrum: Promoting Health and Understanding. *Epilepsia.* 2013;54(2):207–216. doi:10.1111/epi.12056

3. Brodie MJ, Sills GJ. Combining antiepileptic drugs—rational polytherapy? *Seizure.* 2011;20(5):369–375. doi:10.1016/j.seizure.2011.01.004

4. Wiebe S, Blume WT, Girvin JP, Eliasziw M, Effectiveness and Efficiency of Surgery for Temporal Lobe Epilepsy Study Group. A randomized, controlled trial of surgery for temporal-lobe epilepsy. *N Engl J Med.* 2001;345(5):311–318. doi:10.1056/NEJM200108023450501

5. Labiner DM, Bagic AI, Herman ST, et al. Essential services, personnel, and facilities in specialized epilepsy centers—revised 2010 guidelines. *Epilepsia.* 2010;51(11):2322–2333. doi:10.1111/j.1528-1167.2010.02648.x

6. Englot DJ, Ouyang D, Garcia PA, Barbaro NM, Chang EF. Epilepsy surgery trends in the United States, 1990–2008. *Neurology*. 2012;78(16):1200–1206. doi:10.1212/WNL.0b013e318250d7ea

7. Potter JL, Schefft BK, Beebe DW, Howe SR, Yeh H, Privitera MD. Presurgical neuropsychological testing predicts cognitive and seizure outcomes after anterior temporal lobectomy. *Epilepsy Behav*. 2009;16(2):246–253. doi:10.1016/j.yebeh.2009.07.007

8. Ives-Deliperi VL, Butler JT. Naming outcomes of anterior temporal lobectomy in epilepsy patients: a systematic review of the literature. *Epilepsy Behav*. 2012;24(2):194–198. doi:10.1016/j.yebeh.2012.04.115

9. Morrell MJ, RNS System in Epilepsy Study Group. Responsive cortical stimulation for the treatment of medically intractable partial epilepsy. *Neurology*. 2011;77(13):1295–1304. doi:10.1212/WNL.0b013e3182302056

10. Meador KJ, Kapur R, Loring DW, Kanner AM, Morrell MJ, RNS® System Pivotal Trial Investigators. Quality of life and mood in patients with medically intractable epilepsy treated with targeted responsive neurostimulation. *Epilepsy Behav*. 2015;45:242–247. doi:10.1016/j.yebeh.2015.01.012

11. Geller EB, Skarpaas TL, Gross RE, et al. Brain-responsive neurostimulation in patients with medically intractable mesial temporal lobe epilepsy. *Epilepsia*. 2017;58(6):994–1004. doi:10.1111/epi.13740

12. Jobst BC, Kapur R, Barkley GL, et al. Brain-responsive neurostimulation in patients with medically intractable seizures arising from eloquent and other neocortical areas. *Epilepsia*. 2017;58(6):1005–1014. doi:10.1111/epi.13739

13. King-Stephens D, Mirro E, Weber PB, et al. Lateralization of mesial temporal lobe epilepsy with chronic ambulatory electrocorticography. *Epilepsia*. 2015;56(6):959–967. doi:10.1111/epi.13010

Cortical Dysplasia With Extratemporal Epilepsy

Nathan R. Selden

10

Case Presentation

A 6-year-old right-handed female child presents with 2 years of seizures refractory to therapy with methsuximide, clorazepate, and a ketogenic diet, complicated by fatigue related to methsuximide therapy. She has also been previously treated with zonisamide, topiramate, levetiracetam, phenytoin, phenobarbital, oxcarbazepine, valproic acid, clonazepam, and pyridoxine. Since the rather explosive onset of epilepsy at age 4 years, she has never achieved adequate seizure control. There is no history of febrile seizures.

At the time of neurosurgical consultation, she is having an average of eight seizures per day, equally divided between daytime and nighttime. Typical seizures involve leg scissoring, eye deviation, dilated pupils, and a change in level of consciousness. They have already been carefully defined using inpatient video electroencephalography (EEG) monitoring.

Neurological examination reveals a mildly verbally and socially delayed child with normal cranial nerves and a nonfocal general neurological examination.

Medical history is negative, and she does not take any medications unrelated to epilepsy. She has no frank drug allergies.

She has previously undergone 1.5-T brain magnetic resonance imaging (MRI) at age 4 years, which was reported as normal.

Questions

1. Based on her seizure semiology and age, can you formulate a differential diagnosis for the most likely causes of her medically refractory epilepsy?
2. What is the natural history of continued medical and diet therapy, only, for her epilepsy?
3. What is the most appropriate imaging modality?
4. What are the most appropriate electrophysiological and functional tests?

Assessment and Planning

The lack of a history of febrile seizures, auras, epigastric rising, lip smacking, or other classic signs and symptoms of temporal epilepsy points to an extratemporal seizure focus. In a child with no history of cerebral infarct, infection, significant brain trauma, progressive encephalopathy, or other causative event, the most likely diagnosis for the cause of focal epilepsy is a malformation of cortical development (MCD), in particular a focal cortical dysplasia (FCD). FCDs were originally classified by Taylor according to the presence or absence of balloon cells and then more systematically categorized by Palmini. In 2011, the International League Against Epilepsy (ILEA) issued an updated classification, often referred to by its senior author, Blumcke. This classification, refined in 2018, divides FCDs into three types. Type I refers to isolated abnormalities of cortical lamination (radial, tangential, or both). Type II refers to FCDs with dysmorphic neurons (type IIa) or dysmorphic neurons and balloon cells (type IIb). Type III FCD refers to cortical dysplasia adjacent to an early primary brain abnormality: hippocampal sclerosis, glial or glioneuronal tumor, vascular malformation, or other. Type II FCD tends to cause the most aggressive and refractory seizure patterns, but fortunately also responds best to surgery (particularly balloon cell, or type IIb, dysplasia).

The normal MRI obtained in a 1.5-T scanner at a relatively young age does not preclude the presence of cortical dysplasia due to both the immaturity of myelination at this age and the lower sensitivity of 1.5-T imaging. Even when present, cortical dysplasia is often a subtle finding on MRI. Repeated imaging in a 3.0-T scanner using dedicated multiplanar epilepsy sequences and review by an epilepsy program neuroradiologist is performed and reveals an area of likely type I or II FCD in the inferior frontal gyrus (Figure 10.1).

The EEG reveals mild generalized slowing with multifocal independent spike-wave activity, most prominent in the right frontal lobe. Ictal EEG is diagnostic of focal or partial seizures with poor lateralization, suggestive of a deep focus. In light of the failure of EEG to definitively lateralize seizure onset, functional imaging using subtraction ictal single-photon emission computed tomography (SPECT) coregistered to MRI (SISCOM) is obtained to further localize seizure onset. SISCOM demonstrates a likely right inferior frontal focus (Figure 10.2).

Neuropsychological evaluation reveals mild neurocognitive disorder, including significant difficulties with nonverbal problem-solving and reasoning skills.

Oral Boards Review—Diagnostic Pearls

1. Seizure semiology and a detailed neurological examination often contribute critically to accurate localization.
2. Most children who fail adequate therapy with at least two anticonvulsant medications under expert supervision will not become seizure free and will suffer a lifetime of developmental and neurological damage due to both ongoing seizures and the side effects of medications. In such children, epilepsy surgery often offers the only realistic hope for a healthy neurological outcome.
3. Appropriate imaging and functional testing requires leading edge inpatient seizure monitoring, neuroimaging facilities, pediatric neuropsychology, SPECT or positron emission tomographic (PET) imaging, and electrophysiology. Some centers utilize additional testing, including high-density EEG mapping or magnetoencephalography.
4. An expert team in the setting of an interdisciplinary epilepsy board should finalize all surgical planning.

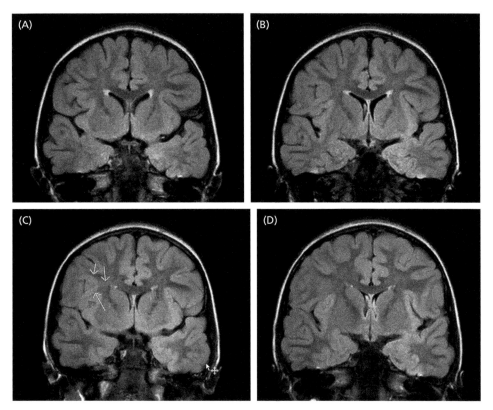

Figure 10.1 Magnetic resonance imaging of the brain at age 4 years (A and B) fails to clearly reveal the presence of right frontal cortical dysplasia, and 3.0-T MRI at age 6 years (C and D) demonstrates the presence of cortical blurring in the inferior frontal gyrus with a deep dysplastic tail extending to the frontal horn of the lateral ventricle (arrows).

Questions

1. How do these clinical, radiological, and physiological findings influence surgical planning?
2. How does the age of the patient influence options for localization and surgical therapy?

Decision-Making

On the basis of these studies, an interdisciplinary epilepsy board, including child neurologists, a specialist neuroradiologist, a pediatric neurosurgeon, a neuropsychologist, and a nurse practitioner, recommend a two-stage surgical procedure for cortical grid and depth electrode implantation followed by hardware removal with likely cortical resection. A two-stage procedure allows a period of days for detailed extraoperative invasive electrocorticography, particularly in children who cannot cooperate with intraoperative mapping. During the interval between the two surgeries, epilepsy medications are weaned to encourage and accurately map the onset zone of resulting seizures. In addition,

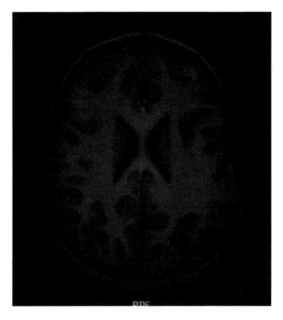

Figure 10.2 Ictal SPECT imaging subtracted from the interictal state (SISCOM) reveals a likely right frontal opercular focus.

adequate time is available for detailed cortical stimulation testing to localize eloquent motor or speech function, even in relatively less cooperative pediatric patients.

The goal of mapping is to identify an area of resection that will offer a high probability of curing the patient's epilepsy and to allow discontinuation of medication without damaging vital neurological functions.

Questions

1. What type of intracranial electrodes should be used for coverage of a lesion with significant representation on the cerebral convexity that also extends to the ventricular ependymal surface?
2. How can intracranial electrodes be safely secured in a younger patient with potentially poor cooperation?

Surgical Procedure

Procedure 1

Implantation of intracranial electrodes is a major procedure carried out under general anesthesia with a Foley catheter in place, duplicate intravenous access, and an arterial line. Given the wide opening and implantation of intradural hardware, brain relaxation is extremely important. Frameless navigation is used to ensure proper location of the electrodes in their intended positions. After fixation of the head in an age-appropriate fixation device and navigation registration, intravenous antibiotics and either hypertonic saline or mannitol should be administered. Hypocapnea, confirmed using blood gasses, should be instituted during the approach.

In the present case, a large bicoronal incision is planned to allow a generous right frontotemporal craniotomy flap. The temporalis fascia is incised in line with the scalp incision, and musculocutaneous flaps are elevated anteriorly and posteriorly. A frontotemporal bone flap is created covering the area of intended monitoring, based on the sphenoid wing antero-inferiorly. A rectangular dural flap is created and rotated anteriorly. Gentle palpation of the exposed frontal lobe reveals an area of slight firmness in the inferior frontal gyrus at the level of the operculum. This area and the area of all implanted electrodes are mapped on a brain diagram by the epilepsy neurologist attending the procedure.

To cover the deep aspect of this lesion, three depth electrodes are placed using stereotactic guidance extending from the surface margins of the dysplasia to near its tip at the ependymal surface. The electrodes are bent at the cortical surface, run posteriorly, and are firmly sewn to the dural edge with an encircling suture. A 64-contact subdural electrode grid is then laid over the exposed cortex and its position confirmed with navigation. The grid is also carefully secured to the dural edges with suture. After closing the dura, the bone flap is replaced over a dural sealant patch, using standard titanium microplates and screws. Four additional screws are placed into the skull, one outside of each edge of the craniotomy flap, away from other hardware so they can be easily recognized on postoperative computed tomography (CT). Each EEG lead is then tunneled to an exit site away from the incision and secured to the skin using a purse-string and roman sandal technique (tied repeatedly after each revolution to prevent slippage). To protect the lead, it is first ensheathed in a 1-inch segment of red-rubber catheter. The dural sealant patch and purse string around each lead exit site are very important to prevent cerebrospinal fluid (CSF) leak around the electrodes and meningitis. The scalp closure is standard.

A CT scan with three-dimensional reconstruction obtained immediately after the first operation rules out the occurrence of a complication or excessive mass effect from the grid and also allows localization of the grid on a reconstructed brain map after fusion with a preexisting MRI. In addition, the CT reconstruction itself can be utilized to register navigation for the second surgery, using the four extracranial screws as internal (highly accurate) fiducials. This is especially useful due to the scalp swelling typically present after the first procedure.

Procedure 2

The patient is returned to the operating room. Setup, positioning, and other preparations should mirror those for the first case. It is not necessary to register the navigation system before the start of the procedure. After the preexisting scalp flap is opened, the four fiducial skull screws placed at the first operation are used to register the fused CT-MRI navigation space. The bone flap is then removed and the dura reopened, taking care to leave all monitoring hardware attached to the dural edges to prevent movement. The electrodes overlying the intended topectomy are mapped out with the neurology team and correlated with adjacent sulcal anatomy. The edges of gyri intended for resection are marked with the bipolar cautery through slits in the grid and then the grid is removed, leaving the depth electrodes in place to help judge the depth of the resection as it proceeds. In certain cases, the edges of the dysplasia are distinguishable from surrounding normal tissue by discoloration or slightly firm texture. The dysplastic tail is followed toward the ventricle and totally resected (Figure 10.3). At our institution, we currently

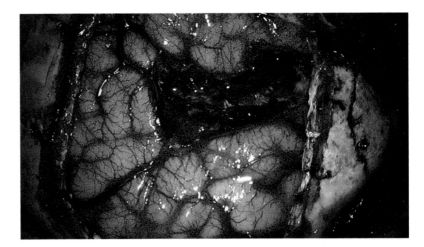

Figure 10.3 An intraoperative photograph shows the focal resection of the inferior frontal gyrus in the opercular region, including the pars orbitalis and pars triangularis.

confirm the extent and depth of resection using intraoperative MRI (iMRI). Closure and recovery are standard. After cutting the leads within the sterile field, the distal portion of each lead should be removed from under the drapes and the exit sites individually sutured following scalp closure and drape takedown.

Oral Boards Review—Management Pearls

1. Total resection of dysplastic tissue significantly enhances the probability of an Engel class I outcome (free of disabling seizures).
2. Resection of type II dysplasia is associated with higher rates of seizure freedom (particularly balloon cell, or IIb, dysplasia).
3. Dysplastic tissue generally follows gyral contours, and resection at the edges of the topectomy should be done using subpial technique.

Pivot Points

1. If noninvasive imaging and functional workup fails to closely localize the suspected seizure-onset zone, or if imaging suggests a focus on the medial aspect of the hemisphere or in the insula, stereotactic EEG (SEEG) may be the best first-stage option to continue the workup. SEEG is useful for identifying the lobe or even hemisphere of onset or to pinpoint very deep foci.
2. If the core seizure focus encompasses eloquent speech, motor, or primary visual cortex, precluding resection, additional nondestructive options may be entertained to provide seizure palliation and medication burden reduction: responsive neurostimulation (RNS), vagal nerve stimulation (VNS), or deep brain stimulation (DBS).

Aftercare

Most patients are nursed in an intensive care unit (ICU) or dedicated neuro step-down unit with specialist nurses and frequent neurological examination. Antibiotics are given for 1 day and a dexamethasone taper for 3 to 5 days after surgery. All anticonvulsant medications are continued after surgery until the treating neurologist elects to taper, typically 3 to 18 months later on the basis of seizure freedom duration and noninvasive EEG monitoring.

Postoperative imaging to rule out complications may be obtained under anesthesia in the iMRI suite or after surgery. We obtain definitive, and final, postoperative imaging 3 months after resection (Figure 10.4).

Complications and Management

CSF leak and meningitis have been described with prolonged grid implantation but are typically avoided with the lead suturing technique described plus meticulous incision closure. Very rarely, a thin subdural hematoma associated with a subdural grid, often with associated cerebral edema, may cause a relatively sudden neurological decline. It is very important in such situations to return urgently to the operating room to remove the hardware and any subdural blood. If mapping is already completed, the planned cortical resection can be carried out early, at that time.

Persistent seizures after topectomy or lobectomy frequently indicate the presence of residual occult dysplastic tissue. Redo invasive workup and further targeted resection may offer the best chance to achieve seizure freedom in such patients.

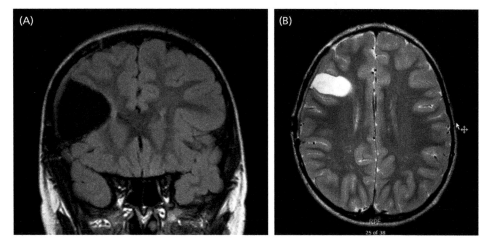

Figure 10.4 Coronal FLAIR (A) and axial T2 (B) MRI showing resection of the inferior frontal gyrus dysplasia, including the entire dyplastic tail extending to the ependyma of the lateral ventricle.

<table>
<tr><td>

Oral Boards Review—Complications Pearls

1. During invasive brain and seizure mapping, patients receiving implants should be observed in the ICU. Any deterioration should prompt urgent imaging and, if necessary, a return to the operating room for hardware removal.
2. Recurrent seizures after multistage intracranial monitoring and topectomy procedures often indicate the presence of unresected dysplastic tissue.

</td></tr>
</table>

Evidence and Outcomes

In large clinical series, seizure freedom is most strongly related to extent of resection of dysplastic cortex, as indicated by imaging and intracranial electrocorticography. Total resection of dysplastic tissue results in seizure freedom in 80% to 90% of patients. Surgery for dysplasia results in seizure freedom in approximately 70% of patients with generally more focal and epileptogenic type II pathology, but only about half of patients with type I pathology. For patients with multifocal or eloquent dysplastic lesions, RNS, VNS, and DBS represent palliative options but provide much lower seizure freedom rates. VNS, the most commonly used, reduces seizure burden in up to 60% of adults and 90% of children, but provides seizure freedom to only a small minority and only while the system is charged and functioning nominally.

References and Further Reading

Alexandre, V, Jr, Walz, R, Bianchin, MM, et al. Seizure outcome after surgery for epilepsy due to focal cortical dysplastic lesions. *Seizure*. 2006; 15(6):420–427.

Gupta, K, and Selden, NR. Cortical dysplasia and extratemporal resections in epilepsy. In Burchiel, KJ, and Raslan, AM, eds. *Functional Neurosurgery* (pp. 129–136). Amsterdam, Netherlands: Elsevier; 2018, in press.

Kim, DW, Lee, SK, Chu, K, et al. Predictors of surgical outcome and pathological considerations in focal cortical dysplasia. *Neurology*. 2009; 72(3):211–216.

Krsek, P, Maton, B, Korman B, et al. Different features of histopathological subtypes of pediatric focal cortical dysplasia. *Ann Neurol*. 2008; 63(3):758–769.

Najm, IM, Sarnat, HB, and Blumcke, I. Review: the international consensus classification of focal cortical dysplasia—a critical update 2018. *Neuropathol Appl Neurobiol*. 2018; 44, 18–31.

Palmini, A, Najm, I, Avanzini, G, et al. Terminology and classification of the cortical dysplasias. *Neurology*. 2004; 62(6, suppl 3):S2–S8.

Taylor, DC, Falconer, MA, Bruton, CJ, and Corsellis, JAN. Focal dysplasia of the cerebral cortex in epilepsy. *J Neurol Neurosurg Psychiatry*. 1971; 34(4):369–387.

Thompson, EM, Anderson, GJ, Roberts, CM, Hunt, MA, and Selden, NR. Skull-fixated fiducial markers improve accuracy in staged frameless stereotactic epilepsy surgery in children. *J Neurosurg Pediatr*. 2011; 7:116–119.

Thompson, EM, Wozniak, SE, Roberts, CM, Kao, A, Anderson, VC, and Selden, NR. Vagus nerve stimulation for partial and generalized epilepsy from infancy to adolescence. *J Neurosurg Pediatr*. 2012; 10:200–205.

Whitney, NL, and Selden, NR. Pullout proofing external ventricular drains. *J Neurosurg Pediatr*. 2012; 10:320–323.

Atonic Seizures

Nathan R. Selden

11

Case Presentation

A 16-year-old boy presents with partial chromosomal deletion, autism, developmental delay, and epilepsy. His epilepsy began at the age of 6 years with progressively frequent and severe tonic and tonic-clonic seizures, associated with moderate cognitive and language deficits. At age 15, he developed additional atonic seizures.

Although seizure holidays were sometimes observed after starting a new medication, his epilepsy was refractory to multiple single- and multidrug regimens, including oxcarbazepine, levetiracetam, zonisamide, rufinamide, and divalproex.

At the time of surgical consultation, he averaged 30 predominantly atonic seizures per day, resulting in repeated injury.

He is motorically normal with a nonfocal neurological examination and is moderately delayed. Cranial nerves are normal. He is normocephalic.

Questions

1. What is the likely diagnosis?
2. What is the most appropriate imaging modality?
3. What additional testing is confirmatory?

Assessment and Planning

The child's primary neurologist assigned a diagnosis of genetically related Lennox-Gastaut syndrome. Lennox–Gastaut syndrome is a severe form of childhood epilepsy involving multiple seizure types, typically including frequent atonic, or "drop," seizures. Intellectual impairment is common.

As in this case, about a third of children, adolescents, and adults with Lennox-Gastaut syndrome experienced a cryptogenic onset. In the other two-thirds, Lennox-Gastaut syndrome may be associated with early or perinatal ischemia, diffuse central nervous system infection, widespread cortical dysplasia, or other underlying etiologies.

Although familial cases do happen, the majority of cases of Lennox-Gastaut syndrome are sporadic. The patient presented here has no family history of epilepsy or other major childhood neurological disorder.

Magnetic resonance imaging (MRI), the primary structural imaging modality for evaluating Lennox-Gastaut syndrome, is typically normal in cryptogenic cases, as it was here (Figure 11.1). Specifically, no areas of brain injury, malformation of cortical

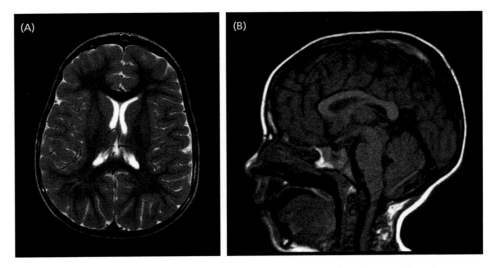

Figure 11.1 (A) Axial T2 weighted and (B) sagittal T1-weighted MRIs showing normal preoperative brain anatomy, including the midline corpus callosum.

development, hydrocephalus, or other abnormality were visualized. There was no hippocampal atrophy or sclerosis.

Electroencephalograms (EEGs) showed generalized slowing with diffuse slow spike wave activity of less than 2.5 Hz.

Additional functional and metabolic brain imaging studies (e.g., single-photon emission computed tomography [SPECT], ictal SPECT, positron emission tomography [PET], functional MRI, etc.) are generally less helpful in evaluating cryptogenic Lennox-Gastaut syndrome.

Oral Boards Review—Diagnostic Pearls

1. Lennox-Gastaut syndrome is a clinical triad consisting of early onset of multiple seizure types (including atonic seizures), developmental delay, and diffuse less than 2.5-Hz spike wave activity on EEG.
2. MRI of the brain is typically normal in cryptogenic Lennox-Gastaut syndrome.
3. Seizure onset may lead intellectual decline by up to approximately two years or vice versa.

Questions

1. How do these clinical and radiological findings influence surgical planning?
2. What is the most appropriate timing for intervention in this patient?

Decision-Making

This patient presents with the classic clinical and EEG findings of Lennox-Gastaut syndrome with cryptogenic onset. In most cases, particularly those of cryptogenic or genetic onset, focal epilepsy resection with curative intent is not possible. In general, there are four categories of palliative therapy for these severe cases of epilepsy.

1. Anticonvulsant medications.
2. Diet.
3. Vagal nerve stimulation (VNS).
4. Corpus callosotomy.

This patient has already proven refractory to years of extensive therapy with anticonvulsant drugs. A ketogenic diet, which may reduce seizure frequency and severity in some patients with Lennox-Gastaut syndrome, was not well tolerated by this patient and his parents. Vagal nerve simulation is palliative for many seizure types seen in Lennox-Gastaut syndrome, but it is relatively less effective for atonic seizures, which at the time of presentation were the predominant seizure type in this case.

Generally, surgical indications in patients with medically refractory epilepsy are determined by an interdisciplinary panel of specialists, often including neurologists, neurosurgeons, neuroradiologists, a neuropsychologist, clinical nurse specialists, and electrophysiologists. In our case, given the limitations of other therapeutic options in this patient, the epilepsy surgery board recommended a corpus callosotomy.

Questions

1. What is the rationale for callosotomy in cases of atonic epilepsy, including Lennox-Gastaut syndrome?
2. How much of the corpus callosum should be transected?
3. What technological adjuncts may be useful for callosotomy surgery?

Surgical Procedure

Atonic seizures result from a sudden, severe, and overwhelming inactivation of both cerebral hemispheres. Transection of the corpus callosum is felt to be effective in treating atonic seizures by interrupting the ability of one hemisphere to synchronously disrupt the other. In children with relatively preserved verbal and intellectual function, callosotomy is often limited to the anterior two-thirds of the corpus callosum, extending roughly to the level of the insertion of the fornix on its ventral surface. This limited callosotomy spares the splenium of the corpus callosum and is relatively less likely to interfere with speech and reading. In children with more limited initial function and in those who responded to an anterior two-thirds callosotomy and then worsened again, a complete callosotomy may be performed.

Experienced surgeons may perform a corpus callosotomy based on anatomical landmarks alone. Certain technological adjuncts, however, facilitate the surgery significantly, even in experienced hands. For example, the extent of an anterior two-thirds callosotomy can be estimated based on physical measurement within the operative field from the rostrum to the posterior border of the transection, comparing the surgical measurement to a preoperative sagittal midline MRI. Alternatively, frameless stereotactic navigation is extremely useful to assess the posterior limit of the transection in real time.

Intraoperative MRI is also useful not only for establishing the extent of the callosotomy, but also for identification of any residual fibers at the inferior extent of the rostrum or postero-inferior extent of the splenium (if relevant).

Callosotomy surgery is carried out under a general anesthetic, with adequate (dual) intravenous access and an arterial line and Foley catheter. The patient is positioned in three-point Mayfield pin fixation with the neck gently flexed and the nose toward the ceiling. I utilize mannitol and controlled lumbar drainage during the procedure to achieve brain relaxation with minimal retraction. Some surgeons tilt the nondominant hemisphere toward the floor to take advantage of gravity retraction, although this may make the angle of surgical attack more awkward.

A limited bicoronal incision is made just anterior to the coronal suture within the hairline, biased toward the right, to facilitate an approach corridor along the right side of the falx cerebri adjacent to the mesial aspect of the nondominant hemisphere. A rectangular craniotomy is planned with 3 cm of exposure on the right and 1 cm on the left of midline, approximately 5 to 6 cm long in the sagittal plane. Two-thirds of the craniotomy should fall in front of and one-third behind the coronal suture. I place pairs of small burr holes at the anterior and posterior extent of the craniotomy, immediately adjacent to the midline, allowing direct dissection of the sagittal sinus dura away from the bone before completing the midline cuts. To strip adherent dura, a single additional burr hole is made on the right lateral extent of the craniotomy at the coronal suture. This bilateral craniotomy flap, extending just across the midline, allows gentle retraction of the falx cerebri, improving the approach corridor. The dura is opened only on the nondominant side, in a rectangular flap based along the sagittal sinus. The length of this exposure allows the surgeon to develop one or two corridors of approach through the interhemispheric fissure around any dominant intervening parasagittal veins. One or two smaller veins may be sacrificed if needed.

Lumbar drainage and gentle progressive intermittent retraction of the hemisphere with suction of cerebrospinal fluid (CSF) from the interhemispheric fissure allow access along the falx. A fixed retractor blade is used without pressure as a guard to protect the mesial surface of the hemisphere while passing instruments. The callosomarginal and then pericallosal arteries are good landmarks prior to encountering the brilliant white surface of the corpus callosum extending in the axial plane. Using navigation, the midline can be confirmed and care taken to dissect arachnoid adhesions between the pericallosal arteries. The pia of the corpus callosum can be lightly bipolared and opened sharply. Suction dissection is generally adequate to transect the corpus callosum, leaving the ventral pia intact (which discourages CSF pressure emanating from the third ventricle). The extent of resection, particularly at the rostrum and splenium, can be confirmed with navigation and, if available, intraoperative MRI (Figure 11.2).

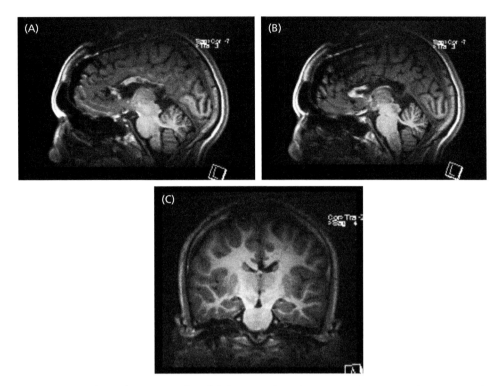

Figure 11.2 (A and B) Sagittal and (C) coronal T1 intraoperative MRIs showing total transection of the corpus callosum. Not that brain shift during surgery prevents seeing the entire corpus callosum in a single sagittal midline image.

Oral Boards Review—Management Pearls

1. Adequate brain relaxation is important to avoid retraction injury to the mesial surface of the hemisphere, which can result in contralateral leg weakness.
2. Fixed retractor blades should only be used to protect the mesial aspect of the hemisphere, avoiding active retraction or kinking of the pericallosal arteries.
3. Using parallax in the sagittal plane, a relatively narrow superficial corridor (between bridging parasagittal veins) can provide access to the entire length of the corpus callosum.

Pivot Points

1. In a patient with higher level verbal, reading, or cognitive function, an anterior two-thirds callosotomy is likely indicated. If seizures improve and then later worsen after a partial callosotomy, the transection can be completed in a subsequent procedure.
2. In a patient with frequent mixed seizure types, including atonic seizures, the initial palliative surgical procedure is often placement of a vagal nerve stimulator. Patients who show improvement in tonic and absence seizures with

VNS but still suffer from frequent or risky atonic ("drop") seizures are good candidates for callosotomy.

3. Many patients referred for callosotomy in the past two decades have had atonic seizures refractory to VNS and were thus ineligible for intraoperative MRI because of the presence of the VNS device.

Aftercare

The lumbar drain and Foley catheter may be removed at the end of the procedure. Patients are nursed for one night in intensive care and then on a dedicated neurosurgical nursing unit. Perioperative antibiotics are continued for 24 hours, and a steroid taper is given for 5 days. All patients should receive a full evaluation by speech and physical and occupational therapy experts. Anticonvulsant drugs should be continued at preoperative dosing levels.

In our case, no seizures were observed for the first 6 months after surgery, likely due to the fact that the patient had been experiencing virtually exclusively atonic seizures immediately prior to surgery. Despite this, his anticonvulsant drugs were maintained at preoperative doses by his neurologist because these levels had achieved near-perfect control of his tonic and tonic-clonic seizure types.

Complications and Management

The patient described in this case experienced moderate new weakness of the left leg and a paucity of voluntary speech, which cleared steadily over a period of 2 weeks. Postoperative MRI showed no cortical injury, ischemia, or complication (Figure 11.3). At 6 months after surgery, motor function was normal, and speech was improved from prior to surgery, likely due to cessation of seizures.

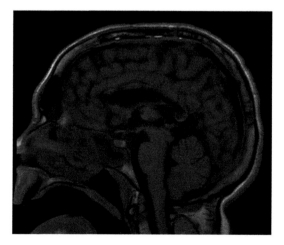

Figure 11.3 Postoperative sagittal T1-weighted MRI shows total disconnection of the corpus callosum without injury to the approach corridor, including the cingulate gyrus.

Transient neurological symptoms are more common after total than partial callosotomy, possibly related to manipulation of a more posterior parietal corridor to complete the splenial transection. Injury to the pericallosal artery resulting in permanent monoparesis is much less common.

Subdural and subgaleal CSF collections are not uncommon after callosotomy but generally resolve without intervention over a period of days to weeks. Hydrocephalus is rare, particularly if the ventral pia of the corpus callosum is left relatively intact. Residual corpus callosum associated with persistent seizures is a risk but is less likely using navigation and is essentially avoidable with intraoperative MRI.

Oral Boards Review—Complications Pearls

1. Recovery is slower and transient weakness of the contralateral leg is more likely in patients undergoing total rather than partial callosotomy.
2. Preserving the ventral pia of the corpus callosum reduces the risk of hygroma and hydrocephalus.
3. Vascular injury is rare but may result in permanent monoparesis of the contralateral leg.

Evidence and Outcomes

Corpus callosotomy is a palliative procedure that is particular effective in ameliorating atonic (drop) seizures. Total seizure freedom after callosotomy occurs in a small minority of patients. Atonic seizure freedom ranges from 50% to 75% and is higher in patients with a normal MRI and in those who undergo a total callosotomy. Seizure medication burden is generally reduced eventually after callosotomy. Complications are relatively uncommon (20% or less) and mostly transient.

References and Further Reading

Camfield PR. Definition and natural history of Lennox-Gastaut syndrome. *Epilepsia*. 2011 Aug;52(Suppl 5):3–9. doi:10.1111/j.1528-1167.2011.03177.x

Chan AY, Rolston JD, Lee B, Vadera S, Englot DJ. Rates and predictors of seizure outcome after corpus callosotomy for drug-resistant epilepsy: a meta-analysis. *J Neurosurg*. 2018 Jun 1:1–10. doi:10.3171/2017.12.JNS172331.

Cukiert A, Cukiert CM, Burattini JA, Lima AM, Forster CR, Baise C, Argentoni-Baldochi M. Long-term outcome after callosotomy or vagus nerve stimulation in consecutive prospective cohorts of children with Lennox-Gastaut or Lennox-like syndrome and non-specific MRI findings. *Seizure*. 2013 Jun;22(5):396–400. doi:10.1016/j.seizure.2013.02.009. Epub 2013 Mar 13.

Douglass LM, Salpekar J. Surgical options for patients with Lennox-Gastaut syndrome. *Epilepsia*. 2014 Sep;55(Suppl 4):21–28. doi:10.1111/epi.12742

Graham D, Gill D, Dale RC, Tisdall MM; Corpus Callosotomy Outcomes Study Group. Seizure outcome after corpus callosotomy in a large paediatric series. *Dev Med Child Neurol*. 2018 Feb;60(2):199–206. doi:10.1111/dmcn.13592. Epub 2017 Oct 23.

Hong J, Desai A, Thadani VM, Roberts DW. Efficacy and safety of corpus callosotomy after vagal nerve stimulation in patients with drug-resistant epilepsy. *J Neurosurg.* 2018 Jan;128(1):277–286. doi:10.3171/2016.10.JNS161841. Epub 2017 Mar 3.

Liang S, Zhang S, Hu X, Zhang Z, Fu X, Jiang H, Xiaoman Y. Anterior corpus callosotomy in school-aged children with Lennox-Gastaut syndrome: a prospective study. *Eur J Paediatr Neurol.* 2014 Nov;18(6):670–676. doi:10.1016/j.ejpn.2014.05.004. Epub 2014 May 22.

Thompson EM, Wozniak SE, Roberts CM, Kao A, Anderson VC, Selden NR. Vagus nerve stimulation for partial and generalized epilepsy from infancy to adolescence. *J Neurosurg Pediatr.* 2012 Sep;10(3):200–205. doi:10.3171/2012.5.PEDS11489. Epub 2012 Jul 6.

Genetic Epilepsy

Nathan R. Selden

12

Case Presentation

A 14-year-old girl with sporadic Rett syndrome, verified by genetic testing, presented to neurosurgery clinic with medically refractory epilepsy. Her seizures began at 6 weeks of life. After a period of remission during childhood, seizures returned and were refractory to medical therapy with valproic acid, clorazepate, phenobarbital, levetiracetam, and topiramate. She experienced tonic, atonic, and partial seizures with vertical eye movements and inattention. Seizure frequency at presentation to neurosurgery clinic was approximately 30 tonic, occasional atonic, and innumerable partial seizures per week.

Neurological examination revealed a developmentally delayed, nonverbal teenager with scoliosis. She followed simple commands and was cooperative and socially interactive. Her cranial nerves were normal. She was tremulous, ataxic, and mildly dysmetric, with a shortened stride length and slow gait, but examination was otherwise nonfocal.

Medical and surgical histories were otherwise negative.

Questions

1. What is the most appropriate imaging modality?
2. What are the appropriate components of the diagnostic workup?

Assessment and Planning

The patient and her parents were referred to neurosurgery by an interdisciplinary epilepsy board for consideration of surgical management. A 48-hour inpatient video electroencephalogram (EEG) obtained as part of the epilepsy workup demonstrated mild generalized slowing, bilateral temporal epileptiform abnormalities, and confirmed seizures.

Oral Boards Review—Diagnostic Pearls

1. Prior to considering surgery for medically refractory epilepsy, EEG or video EEG confirmation of seizure occurrence and semiology is necessary.
2. Typically, patients considering vagal nerve stimulation (VNS) implantation should undergo 3-T magnetic resonance imaging (MRI) to rule out the presence of a focal anatomical abnormality that might represent a treatable source of seizures.

> 3. Potential VNS patients should also be evaluated prior to VNS implantation by an expert epileptologist or epilepsy clinical panel to confirm and recommend appropriate medical and surgical therapies.

Noncontrast computed tomographic (CT) imaging of the brain was normal for this patient, ruling out unexpected complicating factors such as a brain mass, congenital infarct, hydrocephalus, or severe brain atrophy. Because of a confirmed diagnosis of Rett syndrome, advanced imaging such as high-tesla MRI, ictal single-photon emission computed tomography (SPECT), or positron emission tomography (PET) were not undertaken.

Questions

1. Which nonsurgical treatment modalities are available this patient?
2. How do these clinical and radiological findings influence surgical planning?

Decision-Making

In addition to traditional pharmacological therapies, this patient had failed treatment with cannabidiol oil. Some patients with nonfocal epilepsies are also treated with a ketogenic diet. Both of these therapies are typically palliative in this patient population.

Patients with refractory nonfocal epilepsy are generally not candidates for intracranial mapping or resective epilepsy surgery. By contrast, such patients may be excellent candidates for palliative, modulatory epilepsy surgery. The most common technology available in such cases is VNS. VNS therapy is approved by the Food and Drug Administration (FDA) for patients over 4 years of age with partial epilepsy, although equal efficacy has been demonstrated in children with primary or secondary generalized epilepsy.

The VNS systems deliver intermittent bursts of stimulation based on programmed current amplitude, stimulus duration, and interstimulus interval programmable settings. The most recent commercially available VNS system includes a closed-loop feature that allows for the delivery of additional bouts of stimulation in response to sudden cardioacceleration characteristic of seizure onset. VNS systems are generally implanted on the left vagus nerve, which is believed to have a lower risk of cardiac arrhythmia in response to stimulation.

Questions

1. What are surgical contraindications to VNS implantation?
2. How is an appropriate implanted generator chosen for each individual patient?
3. How is lead replacement surgery undertaken?

Surgical Procedure

Surgery is planned to minimize risk of the anterior neck and carotid sheath dissection necessary to implant the stimulator lead. Thus, previous ipsilateral anterior neck surgery and absence of the contralateral carotid artery are considered relative contraindications. Some experts feel that VNS surgical implantation is more difficult, and the risk of surgical site infection is higher, in the presence of a tracheostomy. In all of these cases, VNS implantation by an experienced surgeon is reasonable based on careful analysis of risk and benefit in any individual patient.

The VNS implantation surgery is undertaken under general endotracheal anesthesia, in supine position with a bump under the shoulders and the head resting on a donut ring, extended and rotated about 15° to the right. After administration of intravenous antibiotics, the left neck and chest are widely prepped and draped. I plan a horizontal left paramedian cervical incision about halfway from the sternal notch to the mastoid tip, centered over the medial edge of the sternocleidomastoid muscle (SCM) and the carotid pulse (Figure 12.1). Using an incision at this level, I have encountered no cases of permanent recurrent laryngeal nerve palsy. Some surgeons place the incision two-thirds of the way from the sternal notch to the mastoid, thus avoiding the need to mobilize the omohyoid muscle to reach the carotid sheath.

After opening the incision, the platysma muscle is divided horizontally. The anterior border of the SCM is easily apparent and provides a clean dissection plane leading directly the carotid sheath. The superior belly of the omohyoid muscle may be encountered at the inferior end of the exposure (running, unlike the other anterior neck muscles in the field, from medial to lateral as it courses toward the chest). It may be further mobilized inferiorly as needed. A small curving nerve with one or two branches, the ansa cervicalis, is encountered outside the carotid sheath and should be preserved. The sheath should be opened using sharp dissection along its craniocaudal length, exposing the jugular vein. The carotid artery at this level is just deep to the medial edge of the jugular. In most patients, the vagus nerve is between the carotid and jugular, just deep to the jugular vein. It is larger than the ansa cervicalis and without branches in this segment and should be easy to identify if properly exposed. In a small percentage of patients, the vagus nerve may be more superficial within the sheath. The surgeon should skeletonize about 3 cm of nerve for placement of the VNS electrodes.

For generator placement, I favor a horizontal incision 1 cm below the clavicle. Another option is a vertical incision in the anterior axillary line, which some surgeons feel is more cosmetically acceptable but may be subject to contraction or to infection from apocrine sweat glands. In either case, a pocket is created in the suprafascial plane, generous enough to accommodate generator implantation and layered skin closure without any tension.

The VNS system includes a stimulator lead, generator, and tunneling device. After exposure of the vagus nerve and creation of the pocket, the tunneling device is utilized to pass the lead between the two incisions in the subcutaneous plane, taking great care to pass over the clavicle and thus avoid injury to the subclavicular vessels and apex of the lung. The stimulator lead terminates in three spiral loops, including an anchor (closest to the generator attachment) and positive and negative electrodes. After winding each loop around the vagus nerve, a strain relief loop is created in the course of the lead itself

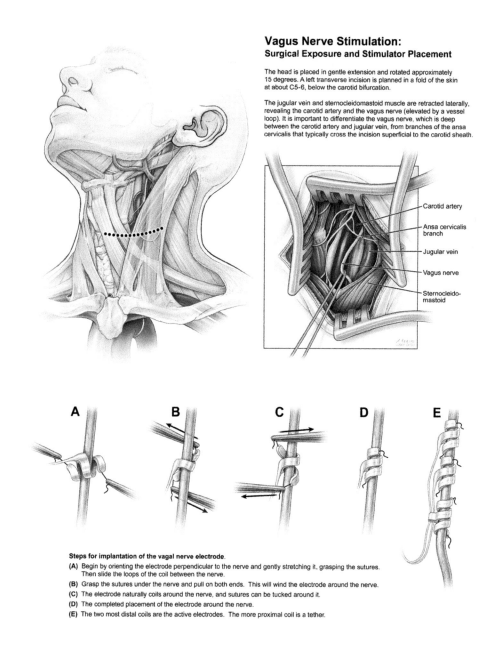

Vagus Nerve Stimulation:
Surgical Exposure and Stimulator Placement

The head is placed in gentle extension and rotated approximately 15 degrees. A left transverse incision is planned in a fold of the skin at about C5-6, below the carotid bifurcation.

The jugular vein and sternocleidomastoid muscle are retracted laterally, revealing the carotid artery and the vagus nerve (elevated by a vessel loop). It is important to differentiate the vagus nerve, which is deep between the carotid artery and jugular vein, from branches of the ansa cervicalis that typically cross the incision superficial to the carotid sheath.

Carotid artery
Ansa cervicalis branch
Jugular vein
Vagus nerve
Sternocleido-mastoid

A B C D E

Steps for implantation of the vagal nerve electrode.
(A) Begin by orienting the electrode perpendicular to the nerve and gently stretching it, grasping the sutures. Then slide the loops of the coil between the nerve.
(B) Grasp the sutures under the nerve and pull on both ends. This will wind the electrode around the nerve.
(C) The electrode naturally coils around the nerve, and sutures can be tucked around it.
(D) The completed placement of the electrode around the nerve.
(E) The two most distal coils are the active electrodes. The more proximal coil is a tether.

Figure 12.1 Steps for implantation of the vagal nerve electrode.

(Figure 12.2), and the lead is then anchored to the muscle fascia with a small plastic anchoring device and permanent suture. At the generator pocket incision, the coaxial pin at the proximal end of the lead is inserted into the generator and secured with the set screw. The generator is then attached to the muscle fascia with a permanent suture. Most surgeons use antibiotic irrigation or powder in both incisions prior to closure. Both incisions are closed in layers with absorbable suture, in watertight fashion to protect the implanted hardware from dehiscence or infection. The key strength layer for the cervical incision closure is the platysma. It is important to "dunk" the lead anchor device under

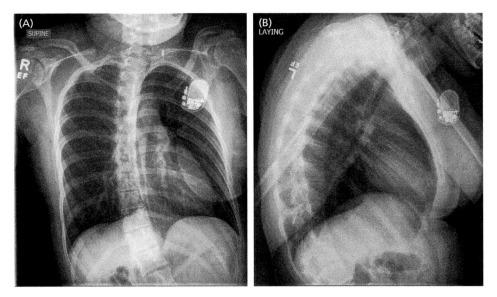

Figure 12.2 A VNS system implanted in the left neck and chest. A strain relief loop is incorporated into the distal lead where the two electrodes and an anchor are coiled around the vagus nerve. (A) Anteroposterior; (B) lateral.

the muscle fascia and secure this covering with suture in order to prevent the occurrence of a subcutaneous lump that is cosmetically apparent.

Prior to removing the drapes, a programming wand draped in a sterile covering is used to test the implanted system for normative lead impedance and function.

The choice of VNS generator for an individual patient depends on size and epilepsy characteristics. Smaller footprint generators may be preferable in younger, smaller patients. Larger generators offer longer battery life, which is important as battery replacement requires surgical generator change.

Lead breakage or malfunction requires surgical lead replacement, which involves a redo carotid sheath dissection. Some centers avoid reexposing the segment of vagus nerve used for the initial lead coil implantation, electing to cut the lead just proximal to the coils. I utilize careful dissection of the existing hardware to reexpose the original segment of vagus nerve, allowing removal of all residual hardware and placement of a new lead on the same portion of nerve. Sharp-tipped Bovie cautery on limited settings may be used carefully to release scar tissue along the plastic sheathing of the VNS system for redo cases.

Oral Boards Review—Management Pearls

1. VNS implantation involves exposure of the carotid sheath and its contents. Meticulous dissection is essential to avoid injury, postoperative hematoma, and airway compromise.
2. Lead impedance and system function should be tested on the operating table to avoid the need for reoperation due to faulty placement, connection, or hardware.

3. Reoperation for total lead removal and replacement on the same segment of vagus nerve, when needed, may be done safely using cautery to carefully dissect scar tissue along the lead's plastic sheathing.

Pivot Points

1. In patients who predominantly suffer from atonic (or "drop") seizures, or those with improved partial but persistent drop seizures after VNS implantation, intracranial surgery for corpus callosotomy may be an effective treatment modality. Prior to the advent of VNS therapy, callosotomy was a frequent intervention for atonic seizures. Although callosotomy is now undertaken less frequently, persistent drop attacks after VNS are currently a common indication for callosotomy. Patients with limited cognitive and verbal function typically undergo complete callosotomy, while others undergo anterior two-thirds callosotomy.

2. Patients with documented cardioacceleration at seizure onset may benefit from implantation of a newer, closed-loop VNS model that delivers additional stimulation in response to the occurrence of a seizure (particularly during sleep, when the patient and caregivers are not available or able to generate an additional stimulation by swiping the generator with a magnet).

Aftercare

Perioperative antibiotics are typically given for 24 hours after surgery. Many centers admit patients for intravenous antibiotics, pain management, and surveillance in case of neck edema or hematoma (which are extremely rare but have the potential to compromise the airway), often using continuous pulse oximetry. However, particularly in adults, discharge after a few hours of postoperative observation is common.

The incisions should be kept absolutely dry for 4 days, after which showering is acceptable. It is imperative that patients not submerge the incisions for 3 weeks to avoid an increased risk of infection.

An early clinic visit about 2 weeks after surgery is undertaken to check the incisions, evaluate for any adverse effects of surgery (e.g., hoarseness), and turn on the system. Definitive postoperative evaluation is usually undertaken at 2 to 3 months after surgery. In most programs, the treating neurologist then follows patients until system monitoring indicates malfunction (e.g., elevated lead impedance or low battery life).

Complications and Management

Recurrent laryngeal nerve palsy is a rare (<1%) but recognized complication of VNS implantation or revision. Persistent hoarseness after VNS surgery should prompt referral to an expert otolaryngologist, who can diagnose recurrent laryngeal nerve injury and mitigate its effects (e.g., with vocal cord injections).

Surgical site infection is another known VNS complication, most commonly occurring in the generator pocket. This diagnosis is made on clinical grounds, with warmth, secondary swelling, redness, firmness, and eventually drainage occurring from the surgical incision, as well as fever and dysphoria. Standard therapy includes immediate surgical removal of all hardware with incision washout and prolonged intravenous antibiotics prior to attempted reimplantation. There are, however, a number of reports of successful lead salvage in the face of generator pocket infection, using a protocol of immediate generator removal, aggressive pocket debridement and washout, intravenous antibiotics, and then new generator reimplantation.

Lead malfunction or low generator battery require surgical hardware replacement, as outlined previously.

The occurrence of transient hoarseness during VNS firing is not uncommon and may occur for a few days or even weeks after an increase in stimulation current. This phenomenon is generally well tolerated and does not cause a failure of therapy, although it may limit current dose in some patients. By contrast, local pain along the course of the lead during VNS firing may indicate compromise of the plastic sheath enveloping the lead, may be associated with impedance changes, and may ultimately require lead replacement.

Finally, serious complications from VNS implantation or revision, while exceptionally rare, may include injury to the vagus nerve, carotid artery, or jugular vein; neck hematoma; and airway compromise. In the event of such an occurrence, complications must be managed urgently or emergently, in conjunction with a vascular or airway surgeon if indicated.

Oral Boards Review—Complications Pearls

1. VNS surgery is generally routine but carries a very small risk of serious complications.
2. Infection and recurrent laryngeal nerve palsy (often temporary) are the most commonly observed complications.
3. VNS-related infection generally requires removal of all hardware and intravenous antibiotic therapy but may be managed in carefully selected patients with a lead salvage protocol to avoid redo neck dissections.

Evidence and Outcomes

Approximately two-thirds of adults and up to 90% of children show meaningful improvement in seizure frequency after VNS implantation for medically refractory epilepsy (generally judged as 50% seizure reduction or greater). VNS also reduces seizure severity, postictal duration, and medication dosing in many patients. In addition, VNS may improve mood in patients with epilepsy-associated depression (and is now FDA approved, independently, for use in some primary mood disorders). VNS implantation early in the course of severe pediatric epilepsy may result in better neurocognitive outcomes.

The use of VNS for medically refractory epilepsy is a palliative therapy. Beneficial effects, which can take weeks or months after implantation to build up, are lost at the time of system malfunction from lead breakage or battery depletion. Even with a fully charged and functioning system, total remission (absence of all seizures) is rare, likely occurring in fewer than 5% of patients.

References and Further Reading

Englot DJ, Hassnain KH, Rolston JD, Harward SC, Sinha SR, Haglund MM. Quality-of-life metrics with vagus nerve stimulation for epilepsy from provider survey data. *Epilepsy Behav.* 2017 Jan;66:4–9. doi:10.1016/j.yebeh.2016.10.005. Epub 2016 Dec 11.

Englot DJ, Rolston JD, Wright CW, Hassnain KH, Chang EF. Rates and predictors of seizure freedom with vagus nerve stimulation for intractable epilepsy. *Neurosurgery.* 2016 Sep;79(3):345–353. doi:10.1227/NEU.0000000000001165

Hong J, Desai A, Thadani VM, Roberts DW. Efficacy and safety of corpus callosotomy after vagal nerve stimulation in patients with drug-resistant epilepsy. *J Neurosurg.* 2018 Jan;128(1):277–286. doi:10.3171/2016.10.JNS161841. Epub 2017 Mar 3.

Ng WH, Donner E, Go C, Abou-Hamden A, Rutka JT. Revision of vagal nerve stimulation (VNS) electrodes: review and report on use of ultra-sharp monopolar tip. *Childs Nerv Syst.* 2010 Aug;26(8):1081–1084. doi:10.1007/s00381-010-1121-2. Epub 2010 Mar 12.

Soleman J, Stein M, Knorr C, Datta AN, Constantini S, Fried I, Guzman R, Kramer U. Improved quality of life and cognition after early vagal nerve stimulator implantation in children. *Epilepsy Behav.* 2018 Nov;88:139–145. doi:10.1016/j.yebeh.2018.09.014. Epub 2018 Sep 27.

Thompson EM, Wozniak SE, Roberts CM, Kao A, Anderson VC, and Selden NR. Vagal nerve stimulation for partial and generalized epilepsy from infancy to adolescence. *J Neurosurg Pediatr.* 2012;10:200–205. doi:10.3171/2012.5.PEDS11489.

Wozniak SE, Thompson EM, Selden NR. Vagal nerve stimulator infection: Lead salvage protocol. *J Neurosurg Pediatr.* 2011;7:671–675.

Focal Spasticity of Upper and Lower Limbs

Walid A. Abdel Ghany and Mohamed A. Nada

13

Case Presentation

A 51-year-old male patient presents to the spasticity management clinic complaining of inability to move his left upper and lower limbs for 1 year. He states that this weakness started acutely with complete flaccidity that progressively improved with time and regular physiotherapy. Now the patient reports that he can independently walk, but he needs assistance during dressing. The patient is known to be hypertensive and has hypercholesterolemia. Detailed neurological examination is done by the multidisciplinary team. The inspection of the left muscle bulk is normal in comparison to the other side. There is hypertonia affecting the left upper limb more than the left lower limb. Weakness involves the distal muscles more than the proximal muscles. The reflexes are exaggerated in left upper and lower limbs. Left ankle and patellar clonus are noted. There is no cranial nerve abnormality.

Questions

1. Define spasticity, dystonia, and rigidity?
2. What is the likely diagnosis?
3. What is the most appropriate investigation you would request?
4. What is the most appropriate anatomical area to image?

Assessment and Planning

Evaluation of a patient with spasticity includes physical, functional, radiological, and electrophysiological assessment. Physical examination of the left upper limb scored II for tone according to the Modified Ashworth Score (MAS)[1] and scored MAS III in the left lower limb. The muscle power in the left upper limb according to the Medical Research Council Scale (MRCS) was graded 2 for finger flexors, 0 for finger extensors, 3 for supinators, 4 for shoulder abductors, and 4+ for the other muscle groups. Muscle power in the lower limb was graded 1 in the tibialis anterior, 3 for hamstrings, and 4+ for the other groups. The patient could walk alone with a circumduction gait. Voluntary movements and selective control of the distal muscle groups were poor in both left upper and left lower limbs. Functional scaling of the left upper limb scored 2 according to the Oswestry spasticity functional scale and scored 3 for the left lower limb.

A magnetic resonance imaging (MRI) study of the brain revealed a small area of right frontoparietal encephalomalacia. A plain x-ray of the left knee joint revealed a high-riding patella (patella alta).

In a conventional nerve conduction study, the H/M ratio was 0.38 for the left upper limb and 0.78 for the left lower limb. Electromyographic recording revealed high spontaneous motor unit activity at rest in all tested muscles.

Gait analysis with dynamic surface electromyography recording for the left lower limb showed out-of-phase activity of the rectus femoris muscle (stiff knee gait pattern). And, there was failure of relaxation of the gastrosoleus complex during the late swing phase (equinus foot).

Oral Boards Review—Diagnostic Pearls

1. The clinical approach to patients with spasticity should be through a multidisciplinary team.
2. The upper motor neuron syndrome (UMNS) results from any lesion affecting the descending motor pathways.
3. The differential diagnosis includes
   - Cerebral infarction: It can be thrombotic or embolic. Major risk factors include atherosclerosis, hypertension, diabetes mellitus, smoking, obesity, and dyslipidemia. In 2013, approximately 6.9 million people had an ischemic stroke, 3.4 million people had a hemorrhagic stroke, and stroke was the second most frequent cause of death after coronary heart disease. Usually, symptoms start with the neurologic shock stage, followed by variable recovery of motor function.[2]
   - Multiple sclerosis is one of the most common central nervous system (CNS) diseases and affects about 250,000 Americans. It is characterized by the appearance of patches of demyelination in the white matter of the CNS, generally starting in the optic nerve, spinal cord, or cerebellum. Most cases occur between the ages of 20 and 40 years. The cause of the disease is unknown, although an interplay between a viral infection and a host immune response may be responsible. It is characterized by attacks (relapses), followed by periods of partial or complete recovery (remissions).
   - Amyotrophic lateral sclerosis (ALS): ALS is a disease confined to the corticospinal tracts and the motor neurons of the anterior gray columns of the spinal cord. It is rarely familial and is inherited in about 10% of patients. The lower motor neuron signs of progressive muscular atrophy, paresis, and fasciculations are superimposed on the signs and symptoms of upper motor neuron disease with paresis, spasticity, and Babinski response. The motor nuclei of some cranial nerves may also be involved. The disease typically occurs in late middle age and is inevitably fatal within 2 to 6 years.

Questions

1. How do these clinical and electrophysiological findings affect treatment planning?
2. Is there a suitable time for intervention in patients with spasticity?
3. What is the value of the motor nerve block test?
4. Describe the stiff knee gait.

Decision-Making

The history, march of the disease, and radiological findings confirm the diagnosis of postischemic stroke left spastic hemiparesis.

Assessment of the left upper limb showed no active wrist or finger extension, with hypertonia affecting the flexor pronator and shoulder adductor muscle groups.

The left lower limb showed weak tibialis anterior action, stiff knee gait with poor foot clearance during the late swing phase, and evident left ankle clonus on touching the ground.

Because this hypertonia was impeding function, the physical therapist referred him to the multidisciplinary team for treatment of the hypertonia.

An important predictor test, the selective motor block test, was performed for the left femoral and tibial nerves. The result of the test was improvement of the ankle clonus and tiptoeing with improvement of the stiff knee during walking (i.e., increased knee flexion angle during the midswing phase of the gait cycle).

The multidisciplinary team decided to surgically reduce spasticity in the left lower limb by selective left tibial and femoral neurotomies and to reduce the spastic upper limb with botulinum toxin type A injection.

Questions

1. What are the phases of the gait cycle?
2. Which would you prefer to do and why: a motor nerve block test or examination under general anesthesia?
3. What is a useful spasticity? Does reducing the muscle tone affect the muscle power?
4. What is the value of dynamic gait analysis?

Surgical Procedure

Examination of the patient under general anesthesia at the start of surgery revealed no contractures in either the left upper or the left lower limb.

Selective tibial neurotomy is indicated for the treatment of varus spastic foot-drop with or without claw toes. It consists of exposing all motor branches of the tibial nerve in the popliteal fossa (i.e., the nerves to the gastrocnemius and soleus, tibialis posterior, popliteus, flexor hallucis longus, and flexor digitorum longus) (Figure 13.1).

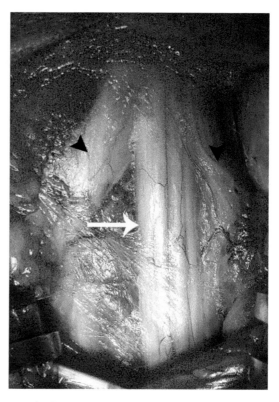

Figure 13.1 Selective tibial neurotomy. White arrow denotes the right tibial nerve main trunk. Black arrowheads mark the motor branches to the medial and lateral heads of gastrocnemius muscle.

The incision can be vertical in the midpopliteal fossa. A transverse incision in the popliteal fossa can be made, which gives a much better long-term aesthetic result. In addition, this transverse incision allows high tenotomy of the gastrocnemius insertion fascia at the end of the operation, if necessary.

Femoral neurotomy is indicated to treat excessive spasticity of the quadriceps muscle. The neurotomy mainly concerns the motor branch to the rectus femoris and vastus intermedius muscles. The incision is horizontal in the hip flexion fold, then medial retraction of the sartorius muscle is done; lateral retraction of the head of the rectus femoris muscle will reveal the femoral nerve trunk just lateral to the femoral artery.

Intraoperative nerve stimulation is essential to differentiate motor branches from sensory branches, especially those of the toe flexors and femoral nerve branches.

Botulinum Toxin Type A Injection

Botulinum toxin is most beneficial in focal and segmental hypertonia. In these cases, it is considered the first-line of treatment because of its low side-effect profile. Most patients experience some benefit within the first 7 to 10 days after injection. Maximum benefit is usually reached after 2 to 4 weeks and then lasts for 12 to 16 weeks. Thus, injections are administered approximately every 3 to 4 months.

Recent practices recommend botulinum toxin treatment as an option in upper limb spasticity or dystonia and state it should be a consideration for focal lower limb hypertonia.[3]

Electromyographic or ultrasound guidance is recommended in these cases to improve the accuracy of injection.

The patient received injections in the pectoralis major, lattismus dorsi, brachioradialis, flexor digitorum superficialis, flexor digitorum profundus, pronator teres, and flexor carpi ulnaris.

Oral Boards Review—Management Pearls

1. The use of an intraoperative nerve stimulator is essential to differentiate different motor branches from other sensory branches to avoid sensory complications.
2. General anesthesia without long-acting muscle relaxation is mandatory to evaluate the motor responses of different branches.
3. Guided botulinum toxin injections give a superior injection result compared to blind injections.

Pivot Points

1. Selective peripheral neurotomy gives a very good and effective long-term reduction of hypertonia in the corresponding muscle group.
2. Patients with progressive hypertonic disorders are not candidates for surgical treatments of hypertonia because of the progressive nature of these diseases (e.g., neurodegenerative disorder).
3. The integration of botulinum toxin type A injections with the other surgical treatments of hypertonia can augment the functional gain for many patients.
4. A regular physiotherapy program and splinting are essential in the postoperative period for optimum results.
5. Selective dorsal rhizotomy (SDR) is the standard technique in treatment of regional spasticity in children with diplegic cerebral palsy. The effectiveness of SDR in poststroke spasticity was documented in a report of two cases in which patients developed unilateral lower limb spasticity.[4]
6. Combined anterior and posterior rhizotomy (CAPR) is a modified technique for management of the mixed spasticity and dystonia by selective cutting of the posterior and anterior roots, respectively, under electrophysiological monitoring of stimulation and recording. It mainly addresses the regional mixed hypertonic conditions.[5]
7. An intrathecal baclofen (ITB) infusion pump enables a higher concentration of baclofen to reach the CNS than can be safely obtained through oral administration. It is particularly efficient in patients with predominant lower limb hypertonia. There have been no prospective studies evaluating its use in patients with stroke. In addition, ITB administration in hemiparetic patients can affect the normal tone or reduce useful hypertonia.

Aftercare

Routine prophylactic perioperative antibiotics are generally given and continued for 5 days postoperatively. Steroids are generally not indicated.

Routine follow-up visits and assessments are scheduled for the first week and first, third, sixth, and twelfth month postoperatively.

Complications and Management

Sensory complications in the form of paresthesias or dysesthesias of the sole could happen. This could be due to neurapraxia of the sural nerve or the soleal sensory fibers traveling through the posterior tibial nerve trunk.

Medical treatments include antineuropathic medications such as gabapentin, carbamazepine, and pregabalin.

The development of secondary resistance to botulinum toxin preparations is an ongoing concern. This could be explained by the development of neutralizing antibodies to botulinum toxin type A.

Oral Boards Review—Complications Pearls

1. Careful dissections and the use of intraoperative nerve stimulation help to avoid sensory postoperative complications.
2. The development of neutralizing antibodies for botulinum toxin type A can be avoided by repeating the injections after a more prolonged period and by using the smallest effective doses.

Evidence and Outcomes

Selective peripheral neurotomy is an efficient neurosurgical procedure in reducing focal and multifocal hypertonia. It can be performed in either upper or lower limbs. Clinical evaluation and motor block testing are very important predictors of the outcome.[6,7]

Botulinum toxin injection of the poststroke spastic upper limb can safely and effectively reduce muscle tone and increase the range of motion.[3]

References and Further Reading

1. Bohannon RW, Smith MB. Interrater reliability of a modified Ashworth scale of muscle spasticity. *Phys Ther*. 1987 Feb;67(2):206–207.
2. Global Burden of Disease Study 2013 Collaborators. Global, regional, and national incidence, prevalence, and years lived with disability for 301 acute and chronic diseases and injuries in 188 countries, 1990–2013: a systematic analysis for the Global Burden of Disease Study 2013. *Lancet*. 2015 Aug 22;386(9995):743–800. doi:10.1016/s0140-6736(15)60692-4
3. Ozcakir S, Sivrioglu K. Botulinum toxin in poststroke spasticity. *Clin Med Res*. 2007 Jun;5(2):132–138. doi:10.3121/cmr.2007.716
4. Fukuhara T, Kamata I. Selective posterior rhizotomy for painful spasticity in the lower limbs of hemiplegic patients after stroke: report of two cases. *Neurosurgery*. 2004;54:1268–1272.

5. Abdel Ghany WA, Nada M, Mahran MA, et al. Combined anterior and posterior lumbar rhizotomy for treatment of mixed dystonia and spasticity in children with cerebral palsy. *Neurosurgery*. 2016 Sep;79(3):336–344. doi:10.1227/NEU.0000000000001271

6. Sitthinamsuwan B, Chanvanitkulchai K, Phonwijit L, Nunta-Aree S, Kumthornthip W, Ploypetch T. Surgical outcomes of microsurgical selective peripheral neurotomy for intractable limb spasticity. *Stereotact Funct Neurosurg*. 2013;91(4):248–257. doi:10.1159/000345504

7. Decq P, Shin M, Carrillo-Ruiz J. Surgery in the peripheral nerves for lower limb spasticity. *Oper Tech Neurosurg*. 2005;7:136–146.

8. Mahran MA, Ghany WA. Spasticity and gait. In: Abdelgawad A, Naga O, eds. *Pediatric Orthopedics: A Handbook for Primary Care Physicians*. New York, NY: Springer Science+Business Media; 2014:375–398.

Intractable Spinal Spastic Paraplegia

Michael Kinsman, Kyle Smith, and Mariah Sami

14

Case Presentation

A 30-year-old male and his wife present to their primary care physician for evaluation of a sacral ulcer that has not healed well despite conservative and surgical treatment. The patient had been in a motor vehicle accident 3 years earlier in which he sustained a complete T7 spinal cord injury (SCI) status after decompression and instrumented fusion at the time of injury. Over the past 3 years, he has managed quite well despite his injury and continues to teach mathematics at the local high school. He and his wife have noticed progressive spasticity in the lower extremities, making it challenging to sit properly in his wheelchair and take care of his perineal region, leading to repeated sacral ulcers and significant pain. He sees a physical medicine and rehabilitation (PM&R) physician, who has been managing the spasticity with oral baclofen with very good results initially; however, with increased dosing over time, the patient has significant medication side effects. He feels that he is having more difficulty concentrating while teaching his students. The patient and his wife feel ready to pursue surgical treatment options. Referral is made to a neurosurgeon.

On detailed neurologic examination by the neurosurgeon, the patient has a T7 sensory level and no voluntary movement below the level of his injury. He is noted to have a suprapubic catheter as he has no useful bladder function. He also endorses bowel dysfunction and is on a bowel regimen that seems to work for him. The patient's legs have significantly increased tone with flexion at the hips and knees bilaterally. Passive movement of the extremities is very difficult, especially with fast manipulation, but can be extended completely with slow manipulation. Examination of the sacral region reveals a stage II ulcer.

Questions

1. Would imaging be helpful in this patient to assist with surgical decision-making?
2. If imaging is warranted, then which regions should be imaged and with what modality?
3. Are the patient's clinical findings more consistent with spasticity or contracture and why?
4. What is the appropriate timing for further diagnostic workup and surgical intervention?

Assessment and Planning

The patient's neurosurgeon suspects that the patient is functionally impaired due to progressive spasticity because of his SCI. Spasticity is a motor disorder that develops gradually after a period of reduced spinal activity and is characterized by increased muscle tone with movement and increased deep tendon reflexes.[1] This increased muscle tone is velocity related and caused by increased excitability of the stretch reflex arc at the spinal cord level.[1] Characteristic postures in patients with spasticity include scissoring of the legs or hyperflexion at the thigh.[1] Spasticity may be painful to patients and may hinder sitting, transferring, lying in bed, driving, sleeping, perineal care, and more. The onset of spasticity after SCI may be delayed for days to several months, often attributed to "spinal shock."[1] Spasticity can provide some benefit if mild. Some benefits may include maintenance of muscle bulk, decreasing the chances of decubitus ulcers over bony prominences.[1] Muscle contractions may reduce the chance of deep vein thrombosis (DVT). Spasticity may be graded using the Ashworth Scale (Table 14.1).[1-3] Assessment of spasticity should be done with the patient supine and relaxed.

The majority of patients presenting to a neurosurgeon for treatment of spasticity already have a clear diagnosis and reason for their spasticity. In our illustrative case, the patient has spasticity due to a complete SCI. Imaging is not usually necessary when assessing patients for treatment of spasticity. One instance where it may be useful to perform preoperative imaging is in a patient who is being considered for an intrathecal baclofen (ITB) pump and the surgeon feels it would be helpful to assess the intrathecal space for possible areas of blockage to catheter advance (Figure 14.1). Other imaging considerations would include preoperative plain radiographs versus computed tomography (CT) to assess bony anatomy, especially if the patient has a history of prior lumbar surgery and an ITB pump is being considered. This imaging may be useful to determine an entry point into the intrathecal space (Figure 14.2). If considering an approach such as a percutaneous radio-frequency rhizotomy, imaging may be useful to determine if the nerves can be approached, especially if the patient is instrumented. In the case of our patient, magnetic resonance imaging (MRI) was obtained and revealed an atrophic spinal

Table 14.1
Ashworth Scale

Ashworth Score	Muscle Tone
1	Normal tone
2	Slight increase with flexion or extension; "catch" felt
3	More marked increase though passive movement easy
4	Considerable increase in tone, with passive movement difficult
5	Affected body part rigid in flexion or extension

From References 2 and 3.

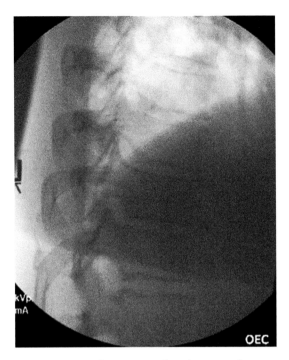

Figure 14.1 Intraoperative x-ray during intrathecal pump placement demonstrating the catheter (with stylet) in the intrathecal space. T10 is an appropriate catheter level for lower extremity spasticity.

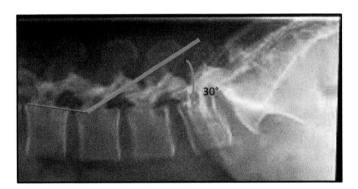

Figure 14.2 A shallow paramedian needle trajectory during placement of the Tuohy needle can minimize complications such as CSF leak and neurological injury.

cord with evidence of myelomalacia at the level of injury and expected postoperative changes for his decompression and instrumented fusion.

Oral Boards Review—Diagnostic Pearls

1. As always, history and physical examination are the most important considerations when evaluating a patient with spasticity, especially regarding distinguishing between spasticity and contractures. This is important because each entity is treated differently. If the patient has significant tendon and

---

muscle contractures and very little spasticity, the procedures we talk about may not provide much benefit, and other approaches should be considered.

2. It is important to document the degree of spasticity with a standard scale such as the Ashworth Scale. This becomes especially important if considering implantation of an ITB pump, where it is very helpful to have documentation prior to undergoing a trial of ITB to compare pre- and posttrial spasticity.

3. Imaging may be helpful for preoperative planning, allowing for informed decision-making regarding choosing a surgical procedure, if different options are being considered. For instance, if the patient has instrumentation or a fusion mass that would make it difficult to access the foramina at various levels or difficult to insert a catheter into the intrathecal space, it may change the planned procedure.

Questions

1. How do these clinical and radiological results influence surgical decision-making?
2. What is the most appropriate time for surgical intervention in this patient?

Decision-Making

Treatment of a patient's spasticity depends heavily on the extent of useful function at the level of and below the level where spasticity begins.[1] Patients with complete spinal cord injuries like our patient usually have very little function, but patients with multiple sclerosis (MS) may have significant function. Most patients are initially managed medically for their spasticity. Medical or conservative management may include prevention of stimuli that would increase spasticity, prolonged stretching, and oral medications. Stretching may prevent joint and muscle contracture as well as modulate spasticity. Oral medications frequently used are as follows:

1. *Baclofen* is a γ-aminobutyric acid (GABA) analogue that binds to presynaptic $GABA_B$ receptors of the Ia muscle spinal afferents, leading to the inhibition of α–motor neurons and ultimately muscle relaxation. It is useful for significant spasticity usually due to SCI or MS. Side effects may include sedation, lower seizure threshold, speech problems, ataxia, confusion, and gastrointestinal (GI) disturbances.[1,3]

2. *Diazepam* potentiates the action of GABA by binding adjacent to the $GABA_A$ receptor, increasing presynaptic inhibition of α–motor neurons and leading to improvement in muscle spasticity. Side effects may include sedation, weakness, and if abruptly stopped, depression, seizures, and a withdrawal syndrome.[1,3]

3. *Tizanidine* is an agonist of the α_2-adrenoreceptor. Side effects may include drowsiness, fatigue, dry mouth, and GI symptoms.[3]

4. *Dantrolene* reduces the concentration of Ca^{2+} in the sarcoplasmic reticulum of skeletal muscle. Side effects include liver toxicity, weakness, sedation, and toxicity in pregnancy.[1,3]

5. *Botulinum toxin type A* inhibits acetylcholine release, providing neuromuscular blockade and resulting in localized control via temporary muscle paralysis. General side effects may include local pain, edema, erythema, and systemic reactions.[4]

Surgical treatment for spasticity is often reserved for spasticity that is refractory to medical treatment or when medication side effects are intolerable.[1] There are two broad categories of surgical treatment: ablative and nonablative.[1] Several of the more common procedures are discussed.

The most common nonablative procedure is insertion of an ITB pump.[5–8] Selection criteria for ITB pump may be found in Box 14.1.[1] Other indications may include traumatic brain injury (TBI), dystonia, stiff person syndrome, cerebrovascular accident (CVA), and cerebral palsy (CP).

The rationale for this treatment modality is that ITB bypasses the blood-brain barrier and allows for appropriate and titratable concentrations of medication at the desired site of action with a half-life of about 90 minutes.[1,3,5–8] A continuous infusion into the intrathecal space provides an antispasmodic baseline. The system components include (1) a pump powered by a lithium ion battery, (2) the intrathecal catheter, and (3) an external programmer that can be used to adjust all settings. The pump typically lasts 4–6 years and is refilled at least every 6 months as this is the typical expiration date of the formulation commonly used.[3] Prior to implantation of the system, patients typically undergo a screening process. This involves a bolus intrathecal injection of baclofen (25–100 μg) with pre- and postinjection assessment of muscle tone and spasticity.[1,3] Patients are typically assessed for 4–24 hours after injection.[1,3] Usually, the daily dose for ITB is twice the test dose per day. Patients should be consented for infection, cerebrospinal fluid (CSF) leak, sedation, headache, constipation, nausea or vomiting, catheter migration, hardware failure, and weight gain.

There are several ablative surgical procedures, including motor point blocks,[9] phenol nerve block, selective peripheral neurotomies,[9] percutaneous radio-frequency foraminal rhizotomy, myelotomies, selective dorsal rhizotomy,[10] stereotactic thalamotomy or dentatotomy,[11] intrathecal injection of phenol, selective anterior rhizotomy, intramuscular

---

Box 14.1 Selection Criteria for Implantation of Baclofen Pump

- Age 18–65 years
- Ability to provide informed consent
- Severe, chronic spasticity due to SCI/lesion or MS
- Spasticity refractory to oral medications or significant medication side effects
- No evidence of CSF blockage on imaging
- Positive response to ITB trial
- No implantable programmable device such as pacemaker
- In females of childbearing age: not pregnant and using appropriate contraception
- No allergies to baclofen
- No history of recent CVA, impaired renal function, or severe GI/hepatic disease

phenol injection, cordectomy,[12] and cordotomy.[1,3] In this section, we briefly discuss a few of these procedures as they are more commonly used.

The indications for selective peripheral neurotomies include medically refractory spasticity localized to a small muscle group supplied by one or a few peripheral nerves that are easily accessed.[1,3] Preoperative motor blocks may be used to simulate the surgical outcome. An example in the upper extremity includes the musculocutaneous nerve in a patient with a spastic flexed elbow. Another example in the upper extremities includes the median or ulnar nerve in patients with a spastic flexed hand or fingers. Examples in the lower extremity include the obturator nerve in patients with spastic flexion-adduction at the hip or the anterior tibial nerve in patients with extensor hallucis spasticity. Appropriate patient selection can lead to good long-term improvement, with significant improvement in Ashworth scores. Patients counseling regarding risks should include infection, CSF leak, paraplegia, sensory deficits, scoliosis, and loss of bowel and bladder function.

Myelotomies such as the Bischof myelotomy involve dividing the anterior and posterior horns via an incision made laterally.[1] This leads to disruption of the reflex arc with no effect on α-spasticity. Midline "T" myelotomy involves interrupting the reflex arc from sensory to motor units without disruption of corticospinal tract connections to anterior horn cells.[1] This procedure has a slightly higher risk of motor function loss.

Selective dorsal rhizotomy is based on work performed over a century ago demonstrating that sectioning of the dorsal roots eliminated decerebrate rigidity.[1,3,10] The procedure interrupts the afferent limb of the reflex arc leading to spasticity. There are several techniques for this procedure, including dividing the dorsal half of each rootlet, performing a functional posterior rhizotomy or sparing one or more rootlet of each nerve root. Use of neuromonitoring during the procedure is advised to ensure elimination of rootlets most involved in the disabling spasticity. Indications for the procedure include children with CP and spastic diplegia or quadriplegia. Adults with spastic diplegia who remain ambulatory are good candidates. After undergoing a selective dorsal rhizotomy, most patients show improvement in motor performance within a few months.[1] The patients counseling regarding risks should include infection, postoperative hematomas, sensory deficits, and motor deficits.

In 1977, Kennemore reported a series of patients with spasticity treated with a percutaneous radio-frequency foraminal rhizotomy with very good results.[13] Small unmyelinated sensory fibers are more sensitive to radio-frequency lesioning than larger myelinated A-alpha fibers of the motor unit. In several studies, the procedure has been shown to be safe and easily performed, with a prospective study showing very good results in patients with posttraumatic spasticity, with an average follow-up of 12 months.[13] The author of the study noted no change in prerhizotomy bowel, bladder, or sexual function.[13] The patient should provide consent for knowledge of general risks of infection, CSF leak, bowel or bladder dysfunction, sexual dysfunction, and general anesthesia risks.

The patient in the illustrative case is a good candidate for several of these procedures. A long discussion with the patient focused on surgical options and risks associated with them. The patient preferred to proceed with a less invasive procedure as he did not want to take much time off from his teaching duties. He also did not like the idea of having to return to the office often for pump refills and was concerned about the risk of hardware failure associated with an ITB pump, maintenance involved, and the risk of baclofen withdrawal. Ultimately, the decision was to proceed with a T12–S1 percutaneous radio-frequency foraminal rhizotomy. Benefits of this procedure include the outpatient nature of the procedure, no significant postoperative restrictions, no need for maintenance of a device or refills, and very good evidence in the literature of efficacy for patients with posttraumatic spasticity.

Questions

1. Why is it important to determine the degree of useful function in the affected areas of the patient's body?
2. Why is it important to understand the patient's bowel, bladder, and sexual function prior to deciding on a surgical approach?

Surgical Procedure

Rhizotomies can be performed in the operating room using fluoroscopic guidance under general anesthesia. A regular operating table or a Jackson table with bumps may be used as long as the patient's spine can be visualized appropriately with the fluoroscopy unit. Patients are positioned prone on the operating table, ensuring padding of all pressure points, especially in patients with contractures. The Radionics (RFG-3c Plus) or Cosman Medical (RFG-1A) radio-frequency lesion generator or similar device may be used for this procedure. The lesion generators are coupled with a thermister electrode and spinal rhizotomy kit (SRK kit). A ground pad is also used for this procedure.

The procedure of Kennemore is then followed, beginning usually at S1 on one side. The patient's paraspinal region is prepped and draped in the usual sterile fashion. The spinal needle is positioned using fluoroscopic guidance at the target neural foramen, and then the electrode is placed through the spinal needle. It is important to consider making stab incisions at the skin entry points for the spinal needle as this allows for greater ease when passing the needle. It is important to ensure that the spinal needle is extradural prior to proceeding with the procedure at each level.

In stimulation mode on the radio-frequency generator, each nerve root is stimulated at 2 Hz, beginning at 0.5 V and increasing to 1.5 V.[1] While stimulating, ensure that the appropriate muscle groups corresponding to the level are activated prior to proceeding with lesioning. Lesioning is typically made at 90°C for 90–120 seconds.[1] This process is repeated at each level, often beginning at S1 and moving up to T12 and is then repeated on the contralateral side. If help is available, you may "ping-pong" back and forth lesioning at each level bilaterally and then move to the next level. An additional step that can be performed prior to moving to the next level is repeat stimulation of the ablated level and ensuring that the stimulation threshold has increased by at least 0.2 V.[1] This ensures that an adequate lesion has been made. The patient's skin is then washed, and if needed, the individual stab incisions may be dressed and closed with Steri-Strips or a stitch as necessary.

Oral Boards Review—Management Pearls

1. When deciding on a surgical procedure for a patient with spasticity, it is important to take into consideration the patient's proximity to the treating facility, the maintenance involved in refilling an ITB pump, and the caretaker's ability to ensure proper postoperative aftercare.

2. It is important to consider the treatment of spasticity prior to considering treatment of contractures because sometimes it may be difficult to determine how much of the patient's symptoms are due to spasticity versus contracture.

3. Though several studies described no significant increase in bowel or bladder dysfunction in patients after performing a rhizotomy, it is important to be aware of the possibility that these important functions may be affected with this procedure, and the patient should be made aware so an educated decision can be made regarding the appropriate procedure.

Pivot Points

1. Extensive instrumentation or bony overgrowth of the lumbar spine on imaging may modify surgical plans in the case of rhizotomy and access to the foramina or in the case of ITB pump placement and access to the intrathecal space.

2. In patients who are good candidates for both rhizotomy and ITB pump placement, the ability of the patient to follow up or the patient's very good bowel or bladder baseline function can steer surgical management.

Aftercare

Postoperatively, the patient is returned to the recovery area until fully recovered from anesthesia. Patients should be instructed to keep the surgical sites clean and dry and to observe closely for signs of infection. Patients may be discharged with diet as tolerated and activity as tolerated. Paralyzed patients need to continue typical skin precautions to minimize skin complications. This is considered an outpatient procedure, so most patients may be discharged home once they meet discharge criteria. It may be reasonable to keep the patient in the hospital if it is felt that instruction should be provided for transfers or ambulation training with the new changes in spasticity afforded by the procedure. Patients may be seen in the office several weeks after surgery to check the surgical site, though this is not necessary because the incisions are quite minor. If no follow-up is scheduled, the patients should be instructed to call with questions or concerns.

Complications and Management

The percutaneous radio-frequency rhizotomy procedure has been shown to be safe, effective, and relatively easy to perform.[1,13–15] The patient should provide consent acknowledging knowledge of general risks of infection, CSF leak, bowel or bladder dysfunction, sexual dysfunction, and general anesthesia risks. In the series by Kasdon and Lathi, there were no postoperative complications, and no patients had a change in prerhizotomy bowel, bladder, or sexual function.[15] This is a major advantage over the use of intrathecal agents or myelotomy. Infections are very uncommon and, if present, are usually superficial infections that can be treated with local wound care or a course of oral antibiotics. CSF leaks are also quite rare and can be managed by observing the patient in the hospital, keeping the patient flat for about 24–48 hours. Another consideration would be a blood patch, if needed. Treating the patient's symptoms while the leak seals itself is very important from a patient comfort standpoint. Bowel dysfunction may require the use of an appropriate bowel regimen and consultation from a GI specialist to determine an appropriate management strategy. As for bladder dysfunction, most of the patients who undergo this procedure already self-catheterize or may have suprapubic catheters. If not, it may be required to place a Foley catheter with consultation of the urology team for management strategies and long-term care.

Oral Boards Review—Complications Pearls

1. Preoperative assessment of bowel and bladder function and monitoring postoperatively will help protect progression of bowel and renal dysfunction.
2. Proper observation and management of patients with possible spinal fluid leak is important from patient comfort and infection prevention standpoints.

Evidence and Outcomes

In 1977, Kenmore reported a series of patients with significant spasticity treated with percutaneous radio-frequency rhizotomy with very good results.[13] A subsequent study by Herz et al. also showed very good results but had a 40% recurrence rate of significant spasticity, requiring a repeat procedure.[14] A more recent prospective study by Kasdon and Lathi revealed very good results in 24 of 25 patients, with an average follow-up of 12 months.[15] In this study, 25 patients with severe spasticity were studied prospectively to assess the efficacy of percutaneous radio-frequency rhizotomy.[15] Most of the prospectively determined goals were met in 24 of 25 patients.[15] No patients in the study had a change in prerhizotomy bowel, bladder, or sexual function.[15] The procedure was found to be very effective in reducing increased tone and reflex spasms associated with spasticity.[15] There was less improvement in range of motion, likely due to preexisting contractures.[15] No patients in the study with preoperative voluntary movement lost motor function; in fact, one patient unable to ambulate preoperatively became ambulatory with the assistance of a cane.[15]

Overall, the presented studies demonstrate that percutaneous radio-frequency rhizotomy is a very effective treatment for posttraumatic spasticity and spasticity of other causes. The procedure is safe and relatively easy to perform.

References and Further Reading

1. Greenberg, M.S., *Handbook of neurosurgery*. 7th ed. 2010, Tampa, FL: Greenberg Graphics; xiv, 1337 pp.

2. Janin, Y., et al., Osteoid osteomas and osteoblastomas of the spine. *Neurosurgery*, 1981. **8**(1): pp. 31–38.

3. Samandouras, G., *The neurosurgeon's handbook*. 2010, New York: Oxford University Press; xxix, 930 pp.

4. Bjornson, K., et al., Botulinum toxin for spasticity in children with cerebral palsy: a comprehensive evaluation. *Pediatrics*, 2007. **120**(1): pp. 49–58.

5. Adler, G.K., et al., Reduced hypothalamic-pituitary and sympathoadrenal responses to hypoglycemia in women with fibromyalgia syndrome. *Am J Med*, 1999. **106**(5): pp. 534–543.

6. Goldenberg, D.L., Fibromyalgia syndrome. An emerging but controversial condition. *JAMA*, 1987. **257**(20): pp. 2782–2787.

7. Hawkins, R.J., T. Bilco, and P. Bonutti, Cervical spine and shoulder pain. *Clin Orthop Relat Res*, **1990**(258): pp. 142–146.

8. Wolfe, F., et al., The American College of Rheumatology 1990 criteria for the classification of fibromyalgia. Report of the Multicenter Criteria Committee. *Arthritis Rheum*, 1990. **33**(2): pp. 160–172.

9. Deyo, R.A., J. Rainville, and D.L. Kent, What can the history and physical examination tell us about low back pain? *JAMA*, 1992. **268**(6): pp. 760–765.

10. Park, T.S., and J.M. Johnston, Surgical techniques of selective dorsal rhizotomy for spastic cerebral palsy. Technical note. *Neurosurg Focus*, 2006. **21**(2): p. e7.

11. Bonney, G., Iatrogenic injuries of nerves. *J Bone Joint Surg Br*, 1986. **68**(1): pp. 9–13.

12. Bell, H.S., Paralysis of both arms from injury of the upper portion of the pyramidal decussation: "cruciate paralysis." *J Neurosurg*, 1970. **33**(4): pp. 376–380.

13. Kennemore, D.E., *Percutaneous Electrocoagulation of Spinal Nerves for the Relief of Pain and Spasticity*. Radionics Procedure Technique Series. 1978, Burlington, MA: Radionics.

14. Herz, D.A., et al., The management of paralytic spasticity. *Neurosurgery*, 1990. **26**(2): pp. 300–306.

15. Kasdon, D.L., and E.S. Lathi, A prospective study of radiofrequency rhizotomy in the treatment of posttraumatic spasticity. *Neurosurgery*, 1984. **15**(4): pp. 526–529.

Dystonia

Zoe E. Teton and Ahmed M. Raslan

15

Case Presentation

The case of a 12-year-old male with a history of glutaric aciduria type 1 (GAT1) complicated by severe tetraplegic dystonia is presented. The patient was first diagnosed with GAT1 at the age of 13 months and was subsequently diagnosed with cerebral palsy (CP) at 3 years of age. He had been slow to meet developmental milestones and at his best was only able to say a few words. Initially, he was able to walk with a walker, but began to regress shortly after the CP diagnosis.

Unfortunately, the patient's mother reports that his condition has continued to deteriorate over the years. She describes issues keeping up with his care and notes having particular difficulty caring for his pressure sores. The patient is restricted to a wheelchair and uses a controlled assistive device while at school. He has had injuries related to his dystonia, including a left forearm fracture after being dropped while being transferred from his chair.

The patient has received Botox injections to all four extremities for a number of years. However, his mother reports that these were not particularly useful and seem to be diminishing in efficacy. His mother also reports that an intrathecal baclofen pump trial was not particularly helpful. Currently, medical therapy includes Artane (trihexyphenidyl HCl), which has been helping his tone somewhat.

Diagnostic brain magnetic resonance imaging (MRI) with fast spin echo recovery T1 sequence shows expected changes of symmetric abnormal volume loss and T2 hyperintensity of the posterior portions of the basal ganglia.

Questions

1. In patients with medically refractory dystonia, what is the most appropriate surgical intervention?
2. What are the surgical target options for surgical intervention?
3. What are the components of a comprehensive dystonia workup prior to consideration for surgery?

Assessment and Planning

An initial history and physical examination will distinguish between dystonia and dystonia plus syndromes; however, they are not sufficient to determine the actual condition etiology.[1] Neurophysiologic tests such as transcranial magnetic stimulation (TMS) and electroencephalography (EEG) are helpful for confirming the presence of dystonia but will

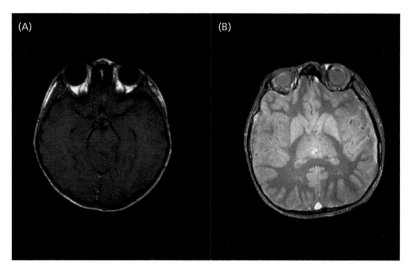

Figure 15.1 (A) MRI with fast spin echo recovery T1 sequence showing expected changes of symmetric abnormal volume loss. (B) MRI T2 showing hyperintensity of the posterior portions of the basal ganglia.

not contribute to etiology identification. Brain MRI may be normal in patients with primary dystonia but can be useful to screen for secondary causes of dystonia (Figure 15.1). Last, fluorodeoxyglucose (FDG) positron emission tomographic (PET) imaging may show increased metabolic activity in the midbrain, thalamus, and cerebellum, but these findings are also observed in asymptomatic carriers; caution is advised when interpreting these results.

Genetic testing should be undertaken to confirm and validate any working diagnosis. This should be done with caution in family members of affected patients as the penetrance of the mutation most often responsible for dystonia (DYT1) is low. In this case, diagnosis was made at a young age and confirmed via genetic testing.

If a decision to proceed with deep brain stimulation (DBS) surgery to treat dystonia is made, a second brain MRI should be used to identify cortical vessels and aid in surgical planning.

Questions

1. Which medical treatments are available to patients that may be tried prior to pursuing surgery?
2. How do efficacy rates compare between stimulation of the globus pallidus interna (GPi) and the subthalamic nucleus (STN)?

Oral Boards Review—Diagnostic Pearls

1. Dystonia encompasses a large, heterogeneous group of neurological conditions, and there is no definitive diagnostic test. It is clinically characterized by abnormal, involuntary, and sustained cocontraction of agonist and antagonist muscles in the body, leading to abnormal posture of the affected area.[2–4]

2. A full preoperative dystonia workup should include a thorough history and clinical examination. Laboratory tests and neuroimaging should be used to rule out metabolic or structural causes. Last, genetic testing, electrophysiological testing, and tissue biopsy may be used to help confirm diagnoses.

3. DBS should be considered once medical treatments either are deemed to be ineffective or are not tolerated due to associated adverse effects or if the degree of disability or the caregiver burden is deemed high enough to consider a surgical intervention.

Decision-Making

Medical management options for patients with dystonia are extensive and will have varying rates of efficacy depending on the type of dystonia being treated. Those most commonly employed include anticholinergics, benzodiazepines, and muscle relaxants. Patients often utilize physical and occupational therapy, and botulinum toxin is commonly used in more widespread cases. Intrathecal baclofen pumps (IBPs) can be surgically implanted as well and are often used, though with varying degrees of efficacy. When considering surgical intervention, there are two decision points involved. The first is whether to pursue surgery, and this should be considered when one of the following has occurred: (1) Medical treatment has been attempted and deemed to be ineffective or the adverse effects outweigh the benefit; (2) when the degree of disability or disease burden is too high for the parent or caregiver to functionally manage; or (3) how prominent pain is as a feature of the dystonia.

The second decision point is that of a surgical target. The most commonly used targets are the GPi and the STN, but both have drawbacks. Historically, the GPi was the most commonly targeted area; however, stimulation here can produce bradykinesia, and often the full benefit of GPi DBS in dystonia is not realized until long after implantation (weeks to months or even years). STN stimulation, on the other hand, has prompted both transient dyskinesia and weight gain in some patients.

For this particular patient, the target chosen was the GPi given that the pathology in this particular dystonia type is known to involve the GPi and given the abundant literature on pallidal stimulation in children.

Additionally, asleep DBS was chosen due to the age of the patient, as well as his prominent dystonic movements. A procedure combining stage I (electrode placement) and stage II was performed under one anesthesia. Image-guided DBS with electrode verification via intraoperative computed tomography (CT) was performed without microelectrode recording.

Questions

1. What are the corresponding target points within the STN and GPi regions?
2. What target error registration error should be aimed for in DBS implantation, and at what error distance should electrodes be repositioned?
3. What are the major complications associated with this procedure?

Surgical Procedure

In the early stages of stereotaxy, microelectrode recording was used to verify that implanted leads were accurately targeted. However, advanced imaging techniques now allow direct visualization of target centers, and they do so in a way that does not require the patient to be awake.

Deep brain stimulation implantation is generally carried out in two steps.[5,6] The first is to place the electrodes themselves, and the second is to implant the internal pulse generator (IPG) about a week later. Prior to surgery, magnetic resonance (MR) images are taken and downloaded onto StealthStation or BrainLab, and surgical planning of electrode trajectories can be done ahead of time. On the day of surgery, once the patient is anesthetized and intubated, the patient's head can be fixed in position using a Halo Retractor System. Five skull-mounted fiducial markers can then be placed and intraoperative CT taken. These stereotactic frame-based CT scans of the brain are then fused with preoperative MR images using either StealthStation or BrainLab.

A nonsterile registration of the previously placed skull fiducial markers will now link the image to the surgical spaces. The predetermined burr-hole entry point should then be marked on the skull with a small pilot hole to identify the intended target. Following sterile preparation, a burr hole is created over the intended site and a second, sterile registration is performed using the implanted fiducials. Target depth is then calculated and placed central to the STN or posteroventral in the GPi with the goal of keeping target registration error less than 5 mm. The dura is then opened, and a cannula is introduced all the way to the target, followed by a DBS lead. The cannula is subsequently retracted and the electrode secured in place using the StimLoc system. A second intraoperative CT scan is then taken to confirm accurate electrode placement. This image is then merged with the preoperative scans, and any error from the target is noted. Electrodes should be repositioned if vector error is greater than 3 mm. The electrodes are then tunneled to a retroauricular area while an infraclavicular pocket is made simultaneously. An extension cable is tunneled, and the battery is connected to the DBS electrodes. Incisions are then irrigated, closed, and then capped.

Oral Boards Review—Management Pearls

1. When performing registration of the scalp fiducials, the operating surgeon should aim for a target registration error of less than 5 mm.
2. Entry point placement should avoid sulci and the lateral ventricles.
3. The coordinates and corresponding target areas within each location are as follows (utilizing the intercommissural plane and midcommissural point for reference):
   a. GPi: Posterior and inferior, immediately superior to the optic tract
      i. Lateral: 18 mm from lateral ventricular wall
      ii. Anteroposterior (AP): 2 mm anterior
      iii. Vertical: 5 mm inferior
   b. STN: Center
      i. Lateral: 12 mm
      ii. AP: 3–4 mm posterior
      iii. Vertical: 4 mm inferior

Pivot Points

1. If the patient in this case were suffering from focal dystonia (affects a single part of the body), a more targeted surgical intervention could have been used, such as myectomy or selective peripheral denervation.

2. If the patient is suffering from more generalized dystonia but would like to forgo DBS implantation, an IBP can be surgically implanted to deliver the muscle relaxant directly into the intrathecal space. This has been shown to be effective, particularly with patients suffering from "spastic dystonia" involving the arms and legs and associated with secondary causes, including tardive dystonia and CP. However, high complication rates and risk of life-threatening catheter leakage decrease IBP utilization rates.

Aftercare

Following the second intraoperative CT scan, no further imaging is required. If this procedure is being performed on an awake patient with mapping, however, a postoperative CT or MRI should be ordered to confirm that the electrodes are indeed in the correct position and confirm that there was no intraoperative hemorrhage (Figure 15.2). The patient will usually remain in the hospital for one night before being discharged the following day. The patient will then return about a week later for IPG placement and can leave the same day following the procedure.

Complications and Management

The main complications from DBS implantation are either hardware-related or due to infection from an implanted device.[2,7] Hardware-related complications include things like lead migration, disconnection and mechanical malfunction, though these are seen in less than 2% of cases. Infection rates requiring surgical intervention range from 1.7% to 4.5%. There is a risk of intracranial hemorrhage at the time of implantation, though

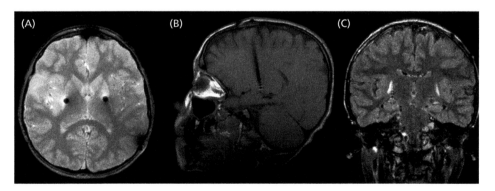

Figure 15.2 Postimplantation MRI showing (A) axial T2 image demonstrating electrode implantation into bilateral GPi; (B) sagittal T1 image demonstrating electrode implantation into GPi; (C) coronal FLAIR image demonstrating electrode implantation into bilateral GPi.

the risk of symptomatic cases is exceedingly low and consistently found to be less than 1.5% in the literature.

Oral Boards Review—Complications Pearls

1. Given that hardware is implanted in this procedure, the risk of infection is inherently going to be higher than that of a lesioning procedure (thalamotomy, pallidotomy). Infection rates can range anywhere from 0% to 15% of cases, but it is difficult to compare due to heterogeneity in what is considered an "infection." For most studies, however, infection rates remain below 3%, with less than half of those requiring reoperation. Infection rates were lowest with consistent surgical teams, strict enforcement of sterility, shorter procedure times, and use of prophylactic antibiotics.[7]
2. While risk of radiographically detectable hematoma is approximately 3% for DBS implants, symptomatic hemorrhages only occur in about half of those cases. This is exceedingly low, especially when compared to the hemorrhage rates in stereotactic biopsy, which are reported as up to 60% in some studies.[8]

Evidence and Outcomes

Dystonia is a lifelong condition that arises from dysfunction of the motor control components of the central nervous system and results in significant pain and disability. It occurs worldwide, and its prevalence varies depending on the classification used. Focal dystonia in the United States affects as many as 30 per 100,000 people, while generalized dystonia affects anywhere from 0.2 to 6.7 per 100,000. Rates are significantly higher in people of Ashkenazi descent, in the population of Northern England, and in the Italian population over the age of 50.[4] Yet, despite its consistent global presence, the pathophysiology of this debilitating condition remains poorly understood. Neuroimaging studies have clearly indicated an association with reduced inhibitory basal ganglia output, failure of cortical inhibition, abnormal integration patterns, and maladaptive plasticity, but a fundamental etiology remains unclear.[3] Most people with a dystonia diagnosis have a normal life expectancy, but the presence and severity of their symptoms are unpredictable and may progress or fluctuate over time. Thus, it is the aim of intervention to improve overall quality of life by minimizing symptoms, increasing volitional motility, and decreasing pain, all while minimizing adverse effects of treatment.

Deep brain stimulation is the primary surgical option for patients and results in varying degrees of efficacy depending on the target location and subtype of dystonia being treated. The GPi was traditionally the target of choice for these cases, but reports of stimulation-induced bradykinesia in initially unaffected limbs has limited use (10 of 11 patients in one study by University of California San Francisco[9]). GPi DBS is also known for taking weeks to months (or even years) to reach its maximal benefit.[2,10] However, GPi stimulation continues to demonstrate symptomatic improvement in dystonia patients with significant reduction in disability (as determined by the Burke-Fahn-Marsden Dystonia Rating Scale disability scale) and improvements in quality of life (as determined by the Short Form-36 scale). The largest prospective study to date followed patients who received bilateral pallidal neurostimulation and found a mean reduction in dystonia severity of 67% at 3 years and 60% at 5 years when compared with their base-line.[11] They also noted that this symptom reduction led to substantial improvements in disability and quality of life metrics, and that these effects were sustained out to 5 years as well. This is consistent with the literature as rates of improvement, ranging anywhere from 60% to 85% in open-label studies and 40% to 50% in randomized controlled trials with at least 6–12 months of follow-up.[2] Unfortunately, these rates are more variable in secondary dystonias and tend to be less efficacious, with improvement rates as low as 20% in dystonia secondary to CP.[12]

While there are generally high rates of symptom improvement in dystonia patients following DBS, there is still a relative paucity of research examining long-term outcomes. Walsh et al. published one of the longest term follow-up studies examining the benefit of bilateral GPi stimulation for cervical dystonia and found that this benefit was maintained out to a mean of almost 8 years.[13]

The STN has only more recently been described as a potential target in DBS for dystonia.[14] While it does avoid stimulation-induced bradykinesia, it comes with an increased risk of dyskinesia and potential weight gain.[2] A 2013 double-blind, prospective, crossover study found no statistically significant difference in efficacy between the two targets in symptom improvement or quality-of-life measures.[6] That same year, another group demonstrated that these symptom reductions and improved quality-of-life metrics were maintained 3–10 years postoperatively (mean follow-up 5.7 years) in patients who received bilateral STN DBS.[15] Overall, both targets appear to be safe and effective stimulation targets in the treatment of dystonia and further study is needed to determine the superiority of one over the other.

References and Further Reading

1. Robottom BJ, Weiner WJ, Comella CL. Early-onset primary dystonia. *Handb Clin Neurol.* 2011;100:465–479.

2. Larson PS. Deep brain stimulation for movement disorders. *Neurotherapeutics.* 2014;11(3):465–474.

3. Pavese N. Dystonia: hopes for a better diagnosis and a treatment with long-lasting effect. *Brain.* 2013;136(Pt 3):694–695.

4. Snaith A, Wade D. Dystonia. *BMJ Clin Evid.* 2014 Feb 28;2014. pii: 1211.

5. Burchiel KJ, McCartney S, Lee A, Raslan AM. Accuracy of deep brain stimulation electrode placement using intraoperative computed tomography without microelectrode recording. *J Neurosurg.* 2013;119(2):301–306.

6. Schjerling L, Hjermind LE, Jespersen B, et al. A randomized double-blind crossover trial comparing subthalamic and pallidal deep brain stimulation for dystonia. *J Neurosurg.* 2013;119(6):1537–1545.

7. Fenoy AJ, Simpson RK Jr. Risks of common complications in deep brain stimulation surgery: management and avoidance. *J Neurosurg.* 2014;120(1):132–139.

8. Binder DK, Rau G, Starr PA. Hemorrhagic complications of microelectrode-guided deep brain stimulation. *Stereotact Funct Neurosurg.* 2003;80(1–4):28–31.

9. Berman BD, Starr PA, Marks WJ Jr, Ostrem JL. Induction of bradykinesia with pallidal deep brain stimulation in patients with cranial-cervical dystonia. *Stereotact Funct Neurosurg.* 2009;87(1):37–44.

10. Petrossian MT, Paul LR, Multhaupt-Buell TJ, et al. Pallidal deep brain stimulation for dystonia: a case series. *J Neurosurg Pediatr.* 2013;12(6):582–587.

11. Volkmann J, Wolters A, Kupsch A, et al. Pallidal deep brain stimulation in patients with primary generalised or segmental dystonia: 5-year follow-up of a randomised trial. *Lancet Neurol.* 2012;11(12):1029–1038.

12. Koy A, Hellmich M, Pauls KA, et al. Effects of deep brain stimulation in dyskinetic cerebral palsy: a meta-analysis. *Mov Disord.* 2013;28(5):647–654.

13. Walsh RA, Sidiropoulos C, Lozano AM, et al. Bilateral pallidal stimulation in cervical dystonia: blinded evidence of benefit beyond 5 years. *Brain.* 2013;136(Pt 3):761–769.

14. Kleiner-Fisman G, Liang GS, Moberg PJ, et al. Subthalamic nucleus deep brain stimulation for severe idiopathic dystonia: impact on severity, neuropsychological status, and quality of life. *J Neurosurg.* 2007;107(1):29–36.

15. Cao C, Pan Y, Li D, Zhan S, Zhang J, Sun B. Subthalamus deep brain stimulation for primary dystonia patients: a long-term follow-up study. *Mov Disord.* 2013;28(13):1877–1882.

Index

Tables, figures, and boxes are indicated by *t*, *f*, and *b* following the page number

For the benefit of digital users, indexed terms that span two pages (e.g., 52–53) may, on occasion, appear on only one of those pages.